ISBN 0-9630738-5-0 $16.95

"Say That Again, Please!"

Insights in dealing with a hearing loss

Best Wishes!

Feby 5, 1992

By Tom Bradford

Published by
Thomas H. Bradford
P.O. Box 12206 — Trust
Dallas, Texas 75225
Atten: Ms. Carol Preston

Book Design by
Susan Neal
Phoenix Design One/Graphic Design
Illustrated by
Michael W. Leone
Photographs by
Tom Gerczynski

Library of Congress Catalogue Card Number: 91-92991

ISBN 0-9630738-5-0

Manufactured in the United States of America

September 1991

10 9 8 7 6 5 4 3 2

First Edition

I would like to dedicate this book to my mother,

Ms. Patricia Wing Pabst,

who never let me know that my hearing loss could have been a limitation.

About the Author

Mr. Bradford was born in Dallas, Texas. He lost his hearing in his right ear shortly thereafter.

He attended public schools in Dallas,Texas; Aspen, Colorado; Orlando, Florida; and LaJolla, California. During his high school years, he attended Culver Military Academy.

He attended Babson College in Wellesley, Mass. where he received his Bachelor of Science Degree in Business Administration with Honors in June, 1972. He continued his business studies at the Babson Graduate School of Business, receiving his M.B.A. with Honors in December of that same year.

After working for two years at the Marine National Exchange Bank in Milwaukee, he returned to college at the University of Northern Colorado, where he received a Masters Degree in Special Education for the Acoustically Handicapped in March, 1977.

He has taught hard of hearing and deaf students for two years in the Corpus Christi Schools, and for five years at the Phoenix Day School for the Deaf.

Currently residing in Scottsdale, Arizona, his outside interests include flying (he formerly flew for an oil company in Alaska, and is a former Flight Instructor), parachuting, scuba diving, and photography.

• • • • • • • • • • • • •

TABLE OF CONTENTS

Introduction

This book was written for the layman. Its purpose is to enlighten those who are interested in learning more about the world of the hearing impaired. It is not meant to be a medical or scientific journal. Every effort has been made to eliminate technical terms.

Chapter One reflects my own personal experiences; the observations and comments are made from my own perspective. I am sure there are others who have had similar experiences and reached different conclusions. I welcome their comments and suggestions.

Chapter Two includes the comments of other teachers and parents. I have found their insights to be invaluable in dealing with this handicap.

Chapter Three contains interviews with several of my former hard of hearing and deaf students. It includes their thoughts about relationships with their families, friends, classmates, and teachers.

Without using medical terms, let me briefly describe my own type of hearing loss. I can not hear with my right ear. Doctors have suggested that there are no longer any nerve endings in the inner ear, which are needed to pick up the sound impulses the middle ear is attempting to transmit to the brain. Since this is true for only one ear, the culprit may have been the mumps virus, which frequently attacks the functions of only one ear at a time. When I was about three I had the mumps, so this is a likely explanation for my hearing loss.

Complicating things further, my left ear has experienced occasional problems since I was twelve. The inner ear would sometimes have too much fluid in it. This fluid would keep the nerve endings in the inner ear from transmitting sounds to the brain in a normal fashion, making sounds harder to hear and distorting them. When the noise level was amplified to make sounds audible, they would suddenly become too loud. This is called recruitment.

CHAPTER I
FROM MY OWN PERSPECTIVE

THE PRESCHOOL YEARS

Diagnosing the Problem

The amount of learning required of a newborn is amazing. The newborn starts out helpless: it cannot identify its own mother or father; it has no instincts that will tell it to fly south for the winter; it cannot walk; it cannot even crawl to find a source of nourishment. With the passage of time and instruction, this will change.

The initial educators are, of course, the parents. They are expected to teach the child everything he will learn until he enters school. At that time society agrees to help with the learning process, for better or worse.

I would like to compare a child's learning process to that of programming a computer, even though a child is considerably more complex than a machine. The parent/teacher will be compared to a computer programmer.

Both the child and computer start out life with a "brain". The child's brain functions normally, and the computer has no short circuits.

We all know that different computers perform differently. Some computers are able to do things that other computers are not capable of, due to the differences in their hardware: the more capacity for processing bytes of information a computer has, the more it can do.

The same is true of humans: different brains work differently. Although size and speed may be factors, there is another element involved.

I submit that one of the most important considerations for both the computer and the child, is the amount and quality of instruction. No matter how large a bank of memory bytes or storage bytes a computer has, if the programmer inserts a poorly designed set of instructions (software) into the machine, then the machine is going to perform inefficiently. It isn't the computer's fault, it's the programmer's.

To a large extent, the same can be said for parents and teachers. If a normal child is not potty trained by the age of six, has no table manners, or cannot read by the time he has graduated from high school, then I suggest the instruction is at fault.

In order for instruction to take place, the pathways of communication must be open. For the purposes of this book, I want to restrict the discussion to the physical pathways (more specifically the hearing/auditory mode), and the insidious, frequently unseen, and potentially devastating results of its impairment.

Let's go back to the computer for a second. How does the programmer get his instruction into the computer? He generally types his messages into the computer on a keyboard.

Imagine if you will, that without the programmer's knowledge, someone rigged his keyboard so that only half of the keys send electrical impulses to the computer. The person who did this little bit of sabotage was clever enough to have all the characters show up on the programmer's monitor. In addition, the computer has no way to warn the programmer of the handicap he is working with. What a surprise the programmer gets when he has given what he feels are good instructions, and his little jewel doesn't do the job.

Please note that only half the keys were made inoperative. The other half are still working. So some response is always noted by our programmer. It would be easier for our programmer to discover something was wrong if the whole keyboard was not functioning, if all the keys were inoperative. He would quickly be able to see there was no response to any of his inputs. Such is the case when a profoundly deaf individual is presented with auditory stimuli.

So the programmer works for hours and hours, day after day, week after week, year after year, trying to teach this "dumb" machine how to do things right. Anxiety mounts; frustration increases. Self-doubt begins to assume a life of its own.

"What am I doing wrong?" says our programmer. "Other programmers are doing fine with their machines."

The analogy of the keyboard and the human ear is fitting. If only half the signals are getting through, then things are going to be frustrating to the programmer/instructor. Neither the computer nor the child knows anything but incomplete signals. In addition, neither the computer nor the child have a way of informing the programmer/instructor (teacher/parent) that there exists a physical impediment.

While it is apparent that something is getting through to the child because there is some change in behavior, the results are not entirely satisfactory. Despite all the best efforts of our instructor(s), progress seems to be painfully slow.

In this situation, a programmer is more fortunate than a parent. After a short period of this nonsense from the computer, our programmer will come to the conclusion that the machine is due for a visit to the repair shop or the garbage heap. The worker at the repair shop will most likely find the source of the problem, declare the machine to be at fault, and for a handsome fee restore the programmer's ego.

Frequently parents are not as fortunate in fixing the problem. You can't see the handicap: the newborn looks perfectly healthy. She will turn her head and look at you. She will look at other objects regardless of whether the objects are making noises or not. She will say "goo-goo" to the dog, the cat, the bird, Mommy, Daddy, and everything else.

This behavior does not mean the child can hear. Even profoundly deaf infants will appear to be acting normally during their first several months of life. It is only months or sometimes years later, depending upon the severity of the hearing loss, that the parents begin to suspect something is amiss.

I would like to emphasize that parents should not be too harsh on themselves for failing to make an early diagnosis. The nature of this handicap is such that even medical experts frequently make mistakes. I am not attempting to excuse incompetence, but the symptoms of this handicap often lead to misdiagnosis. Remember, it is harder to find an error in a keyboard that seems to be functioning correctly part of the time than in one that is completely shut down. It is much more difficult to diagnose a hard of hearing child than a deaf child.

Slow developmental progress has any number of etiologies. Mental retardation is often suggested. There is a host of other possibilities, none of which the parents or doctor can see just by looking at the child.

My own parents did not suspect anything was wrong with me until I was three. One night I went with them to a movie, where I was seated between my parents to insure my safety and good behavior. My father, whom I quickly learned had the power of spankings and therefore had earned my deepest respect, was sitting to my right. Part way through the movie he said something to me and I failed to respond. He said it again a little louder and again I ignored him.

This struck him as being a little odd. He motioned my mother to say something to me, and when she did, I responded immediately. Now I admit I also feared my mother's wrath, but all three of us knew that Dad seemed to be able to elicit the quickest response. Things weren't adding up.

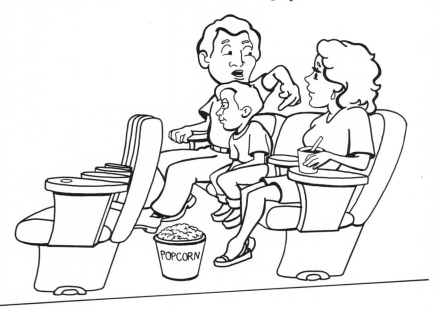

A visit to the local doctor the next day confirmed that their pride and joy was indeed functioning with less than a "whole keyboard." I wonder how long this fact would have remained hidden had it not been for that movie?

Relationships with Parents

Most children are unaware of themselves as being different from others before they're five or six. They simply function as well as they can, whether they are learning to eat, walk, or talk. They know no other standard than themselves. But soon this innocence passes as anxious parents, jealous siblings, and first friends inform the child of his failures, both as an individual and as part of a group. Needless to say, the identity of person making the evaluation, his reasons for making it, and the behavior he is evaluating all influence this judgement.

Evaluating childhood development is tricky at best. Hundreds of books have been written on the subject which give readers an idea of the developmental stages of normal children. Because there are so many variables even for normal children, such guidelines must be viewed as approximations.

Now add a serious complication: the child is able to receive only a part of any instruction given. Frequently the parents of a hard of hearing child don't even know there is a problem. And after the child's impairment is discovered, how do the parents measure progress?

There is just no standard set of guidelines that apply to the development of the hard of hearing or deaf child. The nature of the handicap has so many variables that to use the standards and measures of "normal" development can be very misleading. This is particularly true for developments that require instruction. They are going to take longer. So much for guidelines.

All children want to please their parents, regardless of whether they can hear or not. But if the child does not understand the parents' instructions, then it is going to be very difficult for him to gain their approval.

If you know your child is hard of hearing and you plan to compensate for this by raising your voice, be especially care-

ful of your facial expression. Facial expressions communicate a lot to the hard of hearing and the deaf, but they can
be easily misinterpreted. When you raise your voice, try to
remember to smile!

I recall an incident when I was about four. I was sitting at
our family's dining table. Suddenly I heard my name spoken
in a loud harsh manner. "Oh gosh," I thought, "what have I
done now?"

My father was sitting to my right (remember, my right ear
is for looks only) and was looking at me with a very angry
expression. I was scared stiff. What could I do to make him
happy with me?

It seems he had been telling me the proper way to hold
my fork. I was ignoring him and blithely eating away. I didn't
even know he was talking to me.

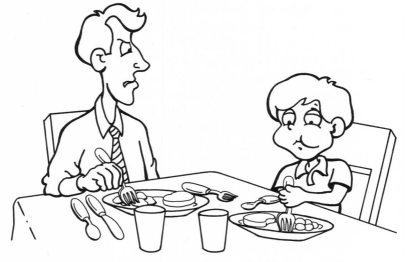

In disciplining their children, parents often raise their
voices and look stern. This usually gains the child's attention.
Be aware though, that this attention does not mean under-

standing. He may know he needs to do something, but he may not know where to begin.

When I was four or five, I didn't know that I wasn't always getting the message. Even when I did get the message, I didn't realize that there was a good possibility that I was only getting part of it. I certainly hadn't learned how to compensate by asking the speaker to repeat his message, or by standing closer to him, or by turning my good ear to him.

When disapproval shows in a parent's face, a child is not motivated to get physically closer to the parent. Parents can very definitely be a source of physical, as well as emotional pain, and a little distance seems like a much safer approach. The look on my father's face did not make me want to stand closer to him and ask him to repeat what he had just said to me!

I agree that parents need to disciple their children and teach them manners, but how this is done is critical. Children want to be physically and emotionally close to their parents, but if their fear of their parents overwhelms this desire, the results can be devastating. A harsh approach will create this fear. The child's solution is to avoid the parents as much as possible. This attitude is easily transferred, as the child attempts to avoid the potential pain of teachers, counselors, and other adults.

This potential withdrawal is magnified with the hearing impaired child. As those looks of disapproval reoccur, the child becomes increasingly wary. It isn't too long before similar looks are received outside the home, and the wariness seems justified not only with parents, but with all adults.

It is important to remember several things about this early period of life. Parents are a child's whole world at this point. Though the child will soon be meeting his first friends outside the family unit, the focal point of learning at this stage is the parents. They set the tone and substance of the child's growth and development. Children with hearing losses are the same as other children. They will laugh, tease, climb trees, and see how much they can get away with.

In my experience, the happiest children are those whose parents have accepted their child's handicap, regardless of its severity. The hearing impairment is never used as an excuse by the parents to avoid discipline. The handicap is also not accepted as a reason for pity from anyone inside or outside the family. This includes the child himself. Duties are shared equally among all the siblings in the family.

Children raised by parents with this attitude develop the confidence to compete with their siblings and go on to cope with the situations that face other children. They attack problems and face challenges without first assuming defeat. Of course, the parents were sensitive to the special needs of these children. These needs were dealt with but were not allowed to assume a life of their own.

Do strive to learn as much as possible about your child's handicap. The more you know about it, the less mystery there is. Be aware of the fact that you are the "programmer" for your little computer. Be sensitive to potential missing information gaps in regard to both learning and behavior. Talk to people who deal with similar situations. Talk to teachers in special education for the deaf, and listen to what they have to say. Most professionals are very committed and can offer sound advice that is not clouded by emotion.

At the same time, do not be intimidated by professionals. Filter the advice that you receive through your own feelings and common sense. You will know your own child because you have spent time with your child. Have confidence in your own perceptions.

In addition, seek out people who can speak from personal experience. Nothing imparts wisdom like experience. No theory or clinical observation can even come close. Talk to other hard of hearing children and adults. Ask their feelings about friends, education, raising a hard of hearing child, and things they find frustrating. Consult other parents of hard of hearing children. Ask them to share their experiences with you.

I believe these two groups - those who have a hearing loss and those who have hearing impaired children - will be your two best sources of practical information and support. You will probably find that many of the experiences and fears that you thought were unique to your situation are shared by others. Knowing this can provide emotional and practical support that is invaluable.

Relationships with Siblings

During these early years, a child's relationships with his siblings depends on a great many factors: the child's position in the family, the number of children in the family, how severe the hearing loss is, how soon the loss is detected, the acceptance or rejection of the child by his parents, the perceived role model for the other siblings to follow, the economic situation of the family unit, etc.

Frequently the oldest child gets the most attention and is the object of the most experimentation in child rearing techniques. This attention can be both a blessing and a burden for the first child, and it is magnified if the first-born is also handicapped.

The blessing is that the first-born enjoys the undivided attention of his parents. The first-born is the fulfillment and confirmation of the dreams of two adults to start a family. Every step is a milestone for both the parents and the child.

This is also a burden. Because this is a whole new game for the parents, they are often anxious and very attentive to the progress of their first offspring. But they have no experience in judging the normal progress of a child's development.

Frequently, the standards that parents set for their first-born are unrealistically high, leading to a high degree of anxiety, wariness, and fear in the child if the parents are not careful.

Whole books have been written about the relationships of siblings, but I do want to raise a few points that pertain to the hard of hearing or deaf child.

The first-born is often the dominant child in a family; being older and stronger, the first-born usually rules the roost. Among youngsters, "older - is wiser - is stronger." If the first-born is not the leader due to a hearing impairment, then what happens to self-esteem?

If parents rely too heavily on younger siblings when delegating minor family chores and responsibilities, then the children will conclude that the hard of hearing child, despite being older, is just not as capable.

Siblings can be quite cruel in establishing a pecking order. Parents need to be aware of the relationships between their children, and particularly between the older hard of hearing child and younger siblings. Allow the hard of hearing child to participate in family responsibilities, discussions, and decision making processes as much as possible.

If the handicap is a severe one, the parents need to take the time to demonstrate compassion for this child. If this is done, but not at the expense of their other children, then the siblings will also develop sensitivity toward their special brother or sister.

As I have said before, the hearing impaired child has no knowledge that he is only receiving part of the intended instruction. He acts upon the information that does get through. This is also true in interactions with siblings.

Back in the days of "Davy Crockett" on TV, when all of us boys wore 'coon-skin caps (that was in the early fifties for those readers who are too young to have had such glory), we always had to have our trusty sidearms. These cap guns made a respectable sound that even I could hear out of my good ear.

I recall a shot going off rather close to me, but I didn't realize it was next to my bad ear. It didn't bother me too much, so I thought I would treat my little sister to some unexpected excitement. Besides, she was a pest. A good scare would do her good! With the proper enticement, she came close enough for me to be able to discharge one of my firearms right next to her ear.

The response was not what I had expected. She promptly screamed and started crying for all she was worth. No gentle words could stop the horrendous noise, and even at that young age I could see that her expression was one of pain. I felt genuinely sorry for what I had done. I had not meant to harm her.

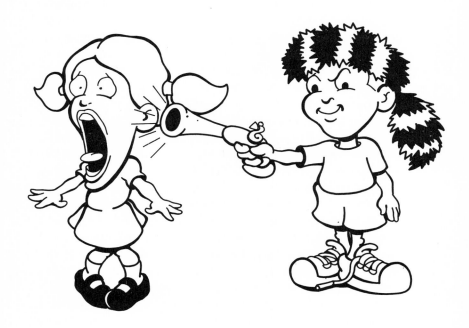

I couldn't understand why she had reacted that way. Perhaps a part of it was the surprise effect of the blast. Maybe a part of it was the disappointment that I would betray her trust. However, the pain expressed in her face was more than these reasons alone would cause. I had the same surprise sprung on me by one of my comrades, but I didn't have any pain. Why did she react differently than I did? It was only many years later that I understood that she experienced what I had missed, the noise and blast of that cap gun.

Relationships with Friends

A child's first friends provide the earliest opportunity for socializing outside the security of the family. A child wants to be liked by others. Learning how to behave, be accepted, and deal with hurt feelings are all a part of this socialization process.

Relating to peers is tough for everybody even when all of a person's facilities are intact. The socialization process is a never-ending process of give and take. It can give a person a chance to develop deep bonds of friendship and trust, and it can also treat one to the agony and pain that comes from betrayals and misunderstandings.

The very first friends a youngster will associate with are most likely other children in the neighborhood. It is important to look closely at these children. It is also important to evaluate these children's parents. Are they the kind of people who are sensitive to the fears and needs of children? If they are sensitive to their own children's needs, then their children are probably going to be just fine as playmates for your child. Interaction with them will most likely enhance, rather than diminish your child's self-esteem.

At this stage, your child is probably still unaware that he doesn't have a fully functioning "keyboard." He will be eager to jump into all the games and activities that other children are playing. Be aware that some of the events you think should be fun are, in fact, loaded with potential confusion for the hard of hearing child. Magnify this one hundred times for the deaf child.

There is so much that is new and confusing to a child at this point that he is not even aware of missing some of the input. He will just figure that the same thing is happening to other children, and that it is normal to misunderstand a lot of things.

During birthday parties when your child does not understand how to play "Pin the Tail on the Donkey," he probably won't be terribly concerned because there seem to be other youngsters who don't understand the game either. And when most of the other youngsters are laughing at something that he doesn't know anything about, he, again, is not terribly concerned: there are other children who aren't laughing either.

He doesn't understand why these other children are not laughing. He doesn't know that it's not because they couldn't hear the funny story: they just weren't paying attention. So the hearing impaired child still feels that he fits in.

Eventually, though, things start to happen that make the perceptive child start to ask questions: Why did everybody suddenly get up and go to the table? How did they know they should move? Why didn't I know that I should be moving with them? Suddenly everybody is laughing. Why? What did I miss that was so funny? I want to laugh, too.

The child soon learns he has to act to appear to fit in. Instead of looking like a fool, he will imitate his peers and laugh at something that is supposed to be funny. He doesn't know what is funny, but at least he looks as though it is funny to him, too. He looks like part of the crowd.

I was unaware that I had a handicap until I was a teenager. When I was a child things happened that left me puzzled. Later, I was able to look back and understand that I had been puzzled because I had gotten only part of the message. Some of these experiences now seem rather humorous, but it is only because they happened in the past. At the time they were anything but humorous.

There will be times that the child will find it easier just to be alone. There are fewer hassles, fewer communication struggles, and less of a sense of not knowing what is going on. By being alone I don't mean a child will sit in a corner doing nothing. I mean he might color in a coloring book. Here is something concrete he has accomplished, on his own, without being bothered by anyone; there are no instructions to follow and no need to get the acceptance or approval of a parent or friend.

Time alone is important. It allows the child to recharge his batteries. When he is ready he will feel like socializing again. Socializing can be stressful when you don't understand why things happen, regardless of your age.

Parents need to realize that there should be a happy medium. Because communication is so much more difficult for the hearing impaired child, there is often a tendency for the child to withdraw socially and emotionally. For this reason I feel it is very important that the hard of hearing or deaf child be given the opportunities to develop friendships with other children who have similar hearing impairments. This is especially important as the child enters the upper elementary, junior high, and high school years.

Language Development

An infant gets his first speech lessons by listening to his parents speak. It doesn't make any difference if the parents are speaking directly to him or not, he is surrounded by the sounds of speech. After several months, given enough input, he starts to imitate these noises: he starts to talk. Initially what he says is meaningless babble, but eventually it becomes clearer.

The child learns that certain sounds convey meaning and that groups of sounds carry specific meanings. He also knows that changing the order of the words can change the ideas conveyed. The child has acquired language. This happens if the child is able to hear: all the keys in the keyboard are working properly. Most of this learning is done before a child enters school. Without formal instruction a child that was initially unable to make a single meaningful utterance, has learned to speak in complete paragraphs in three to five years. Not bad!

Corresponding, the greater number of keys that are not functioning, the greater number of inputs that will be missed. The tremendous amount of learning that normally takes place during in the first four to six years of life will not occur if a child is hard of hearing or deaf.

For example, let's go to watching TV. Let's dial a program that is broadcast in German, but remember, no volume. Now, just how fast do you think you would be able to understand what is going on? How fast do you think you would grasp the meaning of the words? How fast would you acquire the sentence structure of the language? How long would it take you to understand a paragraph? How about idioms such as "raining cats and dogs"?

You say your child is not deaf, only hard of hearing? Okay, let's add a little volume, but let's also turn on the radio at the same volume. Maybe add the dishwasher or the vacuum cleaner. Remember, louder is not necessarily clearer! This

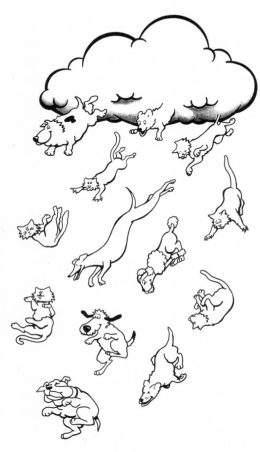

isn't really very much fun, is it?

Now consider that as a child gets older, the rate of learning decreases rapidly. Compare the speed with which infants acquire their native tongue to the years of formal, active study required by high school students when studying a second language such as French or German.

Because hearing impairment blocks early language stimulation, the hearing impaired child runs a great risk of falling behind his hearing peers in language and reading. The earlier a correct diagnosis can be made and corrective action taken, the better for the child. Since early stimulation is so valuable to introduce language, hearing aids and sign language should be used whenever necessary.

If your child can master the language of his society, then the learning process need never stop. Regardless of whether a parent or teacher is present, a motivated individual can always learn new ideas by reading.

Lip Reading

When I am having difficulty understanding a conversation, I will focus on the speaker's lips in an attempt to understand the words being spoken. Sometimes this works, sometimes it doesn't. More often than not it doesn't, but at least I am making an effort.

The idea that someone can tell what another person is saying just by reading lip movements is a fable. The notion that the CIA spy can understand what the KGB spy is saying to his contact on the other side of the room by reading his opponent's lip movements is pretty far fetched.

I realize that KGB and CIA intelligence hardware is capable of doing amazing things and that it is potentially feasible for a computer such as the one in the movie "2001" to understand a conversation between two people just by reading their lips. This could be accomplished by sensing the vibrations of the glass for speech patterns; the vibrations could then be translated into words by the computer. Perhaps some day machines will be able to do this, but human beings are limited in this particular skill.

A certain proficiency can be learned in lip reading. I have met one person who can do this very well. He is exceptional and should be considered such. Insomuch as he is not the norm, anyone who holds him up as an example of what the average person could achieve is simply not in touch with reality.

Let me suggest a little experiment to help you gain an understanding of the difficulty of lip reading. Turn on your favorite TV program. Now turn the volume all the way off. Try to explain the dialogue of the people on the screen to another person in the room. Quite frustrating! (Imagine the frustration of being deaf...)

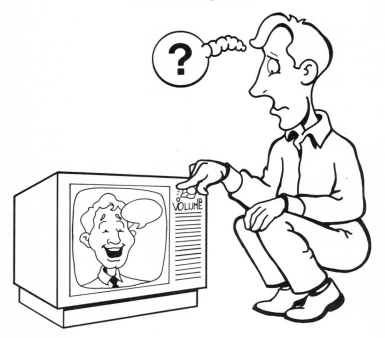

Remember, you have the benefit of your entire education. You know the English language. You know the syntax,
language structure, vocabulary, and idioms. Does your
child?

I am not suggesting that the teaching of lip reading skills
be withheld from those who could benefit from this kind of
instruction. If this same TV had the volume turned up to a
point just short of being able to understand the dialogue
(such as a hard of hearing person might function with the
assistance of a hearing aid), then speech reading would
enhance comprehension. What I am suggesting, is that even
when the listener has had formal instruction, expectations
must be kept in perspective.

Because hearing and speech are so closely related, I would
like to make a few comments about speech development.

The quality of one's speech does not reflect one's intelligence, nor does it reflect the linguistic ability of an individual. Just because I don't understand a Frenchman who is not speaking English does not mean that he is not intelligent!

A balance must be struck in speech training. True, most people in the world communicate by speech; and the better an individual can communicate in this fashion the easier it will be for him to communicate with other hearing people. But not all people with a hearing impairment will be able to develop understandable speech, no matter how many hours they spend studying it. Do make the effort to help your child develop this skill, but be very careful not to give the hearing impaired child the impression that his self worth depends on his ability to communicate orally.

Hearing Aids

"Hearing aids are wonderful little devices that can greatly help to get messages through to the user."

"Hearing aids are often misunderstood and can make the user miserable."

Most people who use hearing aids usually find themselves agreeing at least partially with both of these statements.

I have used hearing aids for several years, both as an adolescent and as an adult. I have also taught and aided classes of the deaf and hard of hearing where these were used with very young children, as well as high school students.

In a nutshell, these devices are not like glasses. With glasses the problem and solution are fairly straightforward. A person is diagnosed and lenses are ground to correct the problem. The correction is usually quite good and consistent in most situations.

Unfortunately, correcting hearing loss is a lot more complicated. It involves more variables than correcting vision. The hearing is impaired, but in what way? Are all frequencies down? Are just the high frequencies down? Are just the low frequencies down? How much loss is there at each frequency? Is the loss equal in both ears?

Another whole set of questions deals with the discrimination of those sounds that are heard. Does the individual understand the sounds that he hears? What do those sounds mean? Just because the sounds are loud enough to get through to the individual doesn't mean that the message is understood.

Hearing aids amplify sounds. One of the problems is that they amplify *all* sounds. Consider the implications of this: if your father's voice happens to be at the same frequency as the motor in the air conditioner, then both his voice and the noise from the air conditioner will be amplified. The listener is then left with the frustrating problem of trying to discriminate between the two amplified sounds. This is no easy task. Add to that all the other noises found in the everyday world: televisions, radios, cars, airplanes, vacuum cleaners, garbage disposals, trash compactors, screaming kids, arguing parents, and you begin to understand the problem.

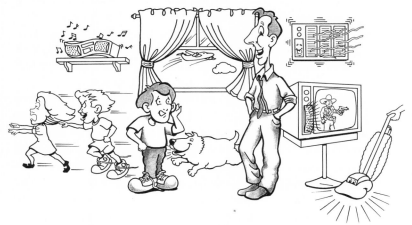

There are seemingly innocent things like the wind. Sounds are received by hearing aids via a tiny microphone. Go outside some day with a regular microphone attached to some amplifying device and plug it into your ears. If there is any wind at all the microphone will pick it up. It can be very loud and distracting. Then have someone stand about five feet away from you and talk to you. Remember the microphone stays with you. Even better, have your friend look away at the same time.

Running water makes noise. Splashing water makes noise. Normal hearing is able to filter out so many noises that most people are not even aware they are present. A hearing aid amplifies all noises so that suddenly even background noises have to be contended with. It is very difficult to understand speech in the midst of all this noise.

In addition, noise and speech sound different through a hearing aid. I can remember many times hearing a noise that I didn't recognize, and then getting up to track down the source of the noise. Usually it was a very common thing - water running in the sink or toilet, a garage door opening, or a furnace turning on. Sometimes it was a somewhat scary noise, a dishwasher suddenly starting a particular cycle or a car without a muffler suddenly zooming by.

The hearing aids made today are designed to address some of these problems: some hearing aids will emphasize certain frequencies over others; some will limit the amount of gain added to an incoming noise, such as the noise of a door slamming. These are great improvements over the earlier aids but there are still many problems involved in using them.

Many times, even with the benefit of a hearing aid, it is a mighty struggle to understand a conversation. When the listener finally gets the gist of the dialogue, it turns out to be trivial: "Aunt Betty's toenail was getting too big for her to wear her pink shoes last week." "I'm straining to hear this!" the listener thinks. It isn't worth the effort.

The hard of hearing and the deaf can be great actors when the effort required is overwhelming. Many times it is so much easier to just smile and nod your head when someone is addressing you. You haven't the foggiest idea of what the person is talking about, but as long as his facial expression is appropriate, you can get by.

I remember many times when I was instructing my deaf students, I would be signing away and watching all those heads nodding, signaling to me that they understood the exciting concept I was presenting. I would then ask one student to repeat what I had just said, and his facial expression would change dramatically: he looked caught.

I must admit that more than once my students caught me doing the same thing to them. They would be talking to me about something and I would be nodding my head. Then they would ask me a pointed question to test my under-standing or to see if I was tuning them out. On occasion they would catch me and we would all laugh as they exclaimed, "Fair! Fair!," meaning it was fair for them to call me on this because I had called them on it. Because we both knew what we were doing, it was fun. We were also signing as well as vocalizing, so the anxiety of trying to communi-cate solely on a verbal level (with or without hearing aids) was missing.

It is hard enough for an adult to try to identify noises and filter out unwanted sounds when using a hearing aid. For a child it is even more difficult and frustrating. I can not emphasize strongly enough the need for caution when putting hearing aids on young children. Children can only depend on adults to do what is right for them. They general-ly want to do what pleases grown-ups. We must be careful not to abuse this trust.

Some of today's hearing aids are extremely powerful: they can knock your socks off. For those children with very pro-found hearing losses they are a great help in getting some sounds through. For some children, though, they can be too powerful. Through audiological testing we are able to make an educated guess about a child's hearing loss. But everyone should be cautious in making assumptions about the accura-cy of the test results in young children.

We also must be cautious when setting the amplification levels of these powerful aids for young children. Parents and teachers must be especially alert to the child's response when using these aids. If the child shows signs of anxiety or nervousness there might be a good reason. It is possible the aid may be set too loud. Nobody likes excess noise thrown at them. A young child without the ability to articulate this problem to you might simply take off the hearing aid. He

might remove the ear piece from his ear or he might resist
your putting it on in the morning.

Try to think beyond his actions to understand why he is
behaving this way. Remember, most children really want the
approval of adults and parents. If he is resisting the use of
the hearing aid at the risk of losing your approval, then
something may be wrong.

If I place a hearing aid in my deaf ear, I can turn up the volume all the way to the highest setting. "Super," one might think,
"now at least I am going to hear something." I get lots of vibrations but not one bit of usable sound. It is something I would
rather do without, and because I am old enough to be able to
say so, I politely decline the use of this much amplification.

But a child is dependent on adults. Very young children
are given aids, and the parent or teacher chooses the amplification on the basis of an educated guess. Please use caution
when doing this.

Energy transfer in fluids can act in strange ways. In one
audiological problem, called recruitment, the inner ear has
too much fluid in it. Sound inputs are impaired and distorted. If amplification is used to overcome the hearing loss, the
increased decibel level can quickly become intolerable. Suddenly the noise is too loud for comfort.

In such cases there can be a real Catch 22 situation: amplification is a possible aid, but only a very specific amount of
amplification. The range of useful amplification is extremely
narrow. If a young child has a hearing problem that involves
recruitment, then amplification of any amount can be quite
bothersome.

Another problem is the discomfort of wearing a hearing
aid. Many people who listen to music have headphones that
wrap around their ears or lay gently on top of them. Not
many people prefer to listen to music by sticking something
inside their ears.

But several factors make it necessary to insert amplification devices inside the hearing impaired user's ear canal. Usually ear molds are custom made to fit the wearer's ear canal. Correctly made, they are reasonably comfortable and many hearing impaired individuals wear their aids all day.

As with clothes that your child outgrows after only a few months, the growing ear canal demands the frequent refitting of the ear mold. Sometimes this must be done as often as every couple of months. Sometimes the mold is not quite right. It is a little too big or a little off on one side. This is very uncomfortable. An adult can protest: "This just doesn't fit right!" But a child often cannot express this. The only thing a child can do is pull the offending mold out of her ear or cry.

A thoughtless parent or teacher might decide that the child is just rejecting the amplification and demand that the child put the mold back in her ear. Please be careful: the child may be saying in the only way she can, "This feels awful!"

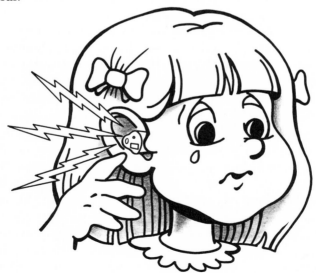

Sign Language

Let's go back to our unfortunate computer programmer. It only makes sense for him to try all the ways he knows possible to get his information into the computer. He will also want to find the easiest method of getting this accomplished.

Likewise, if a child's hearing loss is severe, then alternative methods may be necessary to get the communication pathway open. The use of hearing aids and sign language might be just the ticket.

If the loss is very severe, I implore parents to learn sign language. Its use can bridge the communication gap between you and your child. It is not difficult and can be a lot of fun. It is used by the hard of hearing as well as those who are completely deaf, by older people as well as young. The effort spent now will be repaid many times over. Your frustration level will be greatly reduced. Both you and your child will gain so much by being able to "talk" to each other over the years.

I know whole families who have learned sign language for the benefit of one of their family members. They communicate as a family. They argue as well as laugh together.

I know other families who, tragically, communicate very little with their special family member. At dinner time, while the rest of the family enjoys a conversation about the day's events, the deaf child sits and eats; and for all practical purposes he is alone. The isolation, anguish, and numerous misunderstandings that have occurred over the years, could have been so easily avoided if the parents had accepted their child, handicap and all, and had made the effort to use sign language.

When I was a student teacher, a profoundly deaf high school student entered our classes in the middle of the school year. He had come from a program that did not permit the use of sign language. His lip reading and speech skills were minimal. He was seventeen but could hardly communicate with anyone. He couldn't converse with the other deaf students, and could just barely get his ideas across to the teachers.

When he started to learn sign language, the change was amazing. In a very short time he was able to express his needs and share his thoughts. With the communication barrier broken we were able to get him involved in academic learning. How many years had his learning been delayed? Would he ever really be able to catch up with his peers? And what about his childhood - was he ever really communicating with his parents? Did they know his inner needs and fears?

Other Preschool Thoughts

If my child needed help in acquiring language, I would do several things before he went to school. I would become his teacher and establish a means of communication as quickly as possible. This would involve agreeing on the meanings of words, so as to build a vocabulary base.

Whenever anyone attempted to communicate with him, every effort would be made to control background noise. For example, the house would be carpeted to deaden the sound of footsteps and the banging of furniture. If the house was situated by a noisy street the windows would be closed. The house would be well lit so the child could easily see my face and my lip movements when I was speaking to him. I would make it a point to face my child when I addressed him.

If I felt the loss was severe enough to make auditory learning insufficient, I would use other methods. My house would become a visual dictionary. I would label everything I could with 3 X 5 cards. If I felt it would help, I would learn sign language.

If you get nothing else from this book, please open all avenues of communication between yourself and your child. Life is hard enough when children can hear their parents and can communicate with them. It is so much more difficult when this communication is broken or nonexistent.

Why should any child be locked into a situation where he can not communicate with the people who brought him into the world? Can anybody justify "solitary confinement" at the age of two? That's the effect a severe hearing loss has on a child. Even in the case of profound deafness, sign language can and does break down this barrier. Your child will be forever grateful to you for taking the time to "talk" with him as he grows up.

THE ELEMENTARY SCHOOL YEARS

Role of the Teacher

The first teachers will set the tone for your child's impressions of our educational system. If self-esteem, confidence, and success are encouraged by the teachers, then the child will feel good about himself and this game of education. Children naturally want to please adults, so this gives teachers a bit of a head start. The hope is that this head start is not squandered.

Although teaching is a difficult and sometimes unrewarding job, society is blessed with people who do choose to enter and remain in this profession. The good ones remain for the love of children. When you find a good teacher, cherish him or her. Teachers often devote a great deal to their charges, and many become exhausted in five years.

Occasionally you will run into another kind of teacher: the kind that wants to get out of the profession but can't. They are people who have mortgages to pay, so they stay and cope. They are tired and really don't want to teach anymore. This is sad because they influence children. They are not sympathetic when your child feels hurt; they are not patient; they often don't encourage success. Fortunately this type of teacher is in the minority.

What does a parent do about his child's formal education? Get to know your child's teachers. This means repeatedly going in and talking with the teachers. Ascertain what their goals are for your child. Good teachers will welcome this as a sign of an interested parent.

Talk to the teacher's principal. Get a feel for what direction he has for the school. If he has no real direction, that will tell you something about the school.

Talk to other people in the school administration. What are their goals for the children? How do they evaluate those goals? If a child does not seem to be making progress, what concrete plans does the administration have for giving the child extra help? Are these plans willingly and aggressively provided for, or does the parent have to plead for assistance?

Constantly monitor what kind of work your child is doing in school. When your child comes home from school, do you always seem to have to teach the school work again? Occasional help is one thing, but three nights out of five, every week, is reason for concern: either the child is in the wrong class or the teacher is not teaching the subject. What kind of homework is your child bringing home? Doesn't he ever have any homework? Then I would question whether the child is being challenged, even in elementary school. I strongly believe that the child, who never has homework during his junior and senior high school years, is not being properly taught.

You are the ultimate judge of what is happening. Trust your feelings. If you are not satisfied, then do whatever is necessary to move your child out of the situation.

I think most students in deaf schools are there precisely because they could not cope with the pace of instruction given in the regular classroom. Returning them to a regular classroom would not necessarily help them academically, and would certainly isolate them socially.

The best solution is to bring up the standards of the deaf schools. This has to be done at all grade levels. You can't suddenly impose high standards in the ninth grade. A student that has been passed year after year without achieving set standards at appropriate grade levels has not been well served. If a student does not make the grade for that grade level then he should not be passed. Are we really doing our children any favors when we give them diplomas, but they can't read at the fourth grade level or do third grade math? I think this borders on educational fraud, and it is currently being conducted on a massive scale. I might add that I don't think schools for the deaf have a monopoly on this sorry state of affairs.

Do not accept "sweet-talk." If you feel your child's best interests are not being met, change schools if you have to. Remember, this is your child, not the school's child.

In evaluating a teacher for a hard of hearing child, be especially alert to several things. Does the teacher maintain control of the class? When instruction is being given, does all other student conversation cease? It is extremely difficult for a hard of hearing person to block out one conversation and concentrate on another. If the teacher is in control, then only one person should be talking at a time.

Does the teacher face the class when she is addressing the students? Some teachers talk to the chalk board as they explain. This makes it very difficult for the hard of hearing student to understand.

Are you able to convey to the teacher that your hard of hearing child's ability to hear will appear to vary from time to time? There will be times when she will seem to hear very well, and other times when she does not seem to be receiving any input at all.

Many people interpret this variance as the result of the selective hearing done by the student: she hears when she wants to hear, and tunes out when she doesn't want to participate. Be careful of rushing to this conclusion. There are situations when I can hear and understand the conversation quite well, but there are other times when I find it almost impossible to follow what is being said.

Some people have told me that they think I have been selective in some situations, but the reality is that I could not hear. Background music or noise, the speaker standing on my deaf side, a woman's or child's high pitched voice, and multiple conversations all make it hard for me to follow a specific dialogue.

By talking with your child's teacher, you should be able to detect whether the teacher is receptive to having a hard of hearing student in the class. Most teachers will do everything they can to learn about how they can help your child.

At the same time be aware that if there are thirty or more students in this class, the teacher's ability to give your child individual attention is limited. Understand that the teacher is only human, and that school systems frequently make impossible demands on teachers. They do the best they can with the time and resources at their disposal.

Use common sense in evaluating your child's teacher. Demand high standards, but temper this with the knowledge that most teachers are doing their best. Ideally, the education of your child will involve teamwork: both parents and teachers must be willing to accept responsibility. Educating the hard of hearing or deaf child involves the home as well as the school. Neither can do a good job independent of the other.

The Classroom Environment

The classroom teacher may not have had any experience in dealing with a hard of hearing child, but inexperience shouldn't cause parental panic. If the teacher is good, she will be receptive to your suggestions. She will do all that is humanly possible to help your child, given the situation she has to deal with, such as having 30 or more students in the classroom.

In discussions with the teacher, do not hide your child's hearing loss. The more knowledge and education the teacher has when dealing with your child, the more she can respond to your child's needs.

Is the room well lit? Can the teacher's face and lips be easily seen by the student? If one side of the classroom has a window, then position the hearing impaired student so she does not have to fight the glare.

During my early school years, my mother always talked with my teachers without my knowledge. At the start of every school year when desk assignments were made, I was always assigned a front row seat on the right side of the classroom.

I liked the front row because that was where all the action was taking place. It wasn't until much later in life that I realized these placements were the result of my mother's discussions with my teachers.

Request that your child be assigned to a front row seat. The closer she is to the voice of the teacher the better she will be able to understand.

In addition, if your child has a loss in only one ear, say her right ear, then further request that her seating assignment be in the right front row of the classroom. In this position, her left ear will be facing the rest of the class. She will be able to better understand classroom discussions.

Listen closely to the noise level. Noise that interferes with instruction comes in various, and sometimes insidious forms:

a loud fan in the room will not help, nor will construction near the classroom, nor will a busy street. Is the door to the hallway closed to keep out noise?

Is the classroom an open classroom? If so, it may be divided into learning centers. These can function as noise centers with no physical walls to keep the noise in one area from drifting into another area. This may only be somewhat distracting for hearing students, but it can create an almost impossible situation for the hard of hearing child. Some type of walls or barriers would be a great help.

What kind of floor does the classroom have? Carpeting is a great aid in muffling the sounds of scuffling feet and the moving of chairs and desks.

Classmates

It is during the first years in school a child usually becomes aware that he is different from others. His reactions to situations will be different than those of his classmates, and he will be consciously aware of these differences for the first time. Sometimes hurt arises because the child is in situation he does not understand. This frequently occurs when a child is hard of hearing or deaf.

What follows are several examples. I think they are probably typical of what many children have to go through during these years, but the situations were compounded by difficulties that come with being hard of hearing.

When I was in first grade, the school patrol came into the classroom and told the teacher and the class that I was not riding my bicycle to school on the correct side of the road. I was mortified. I didn't want these older schoolmates and my own classmates to think I was a fool.

I was told that I should ride my bicycle on the other side of the road. The next day I made a point of riding on the other side of the road, taking great pride in doing what was right.

Suddenly, just before school started, the patrol appeared again. I was wrong again. I must have heard incorrectly. I would change again, and do it the other way. I was sorry.

The third day I was confused. There was only two sides of the street. Which one was correct? I elected to take the one I tried two days ago, since yesterday's route was the most recent error.

They came back again! My frustration was unloaded in tears. I was trying to do what was right, but I didn't understand.

The teacher drew the approach I should have taken on the blackboard. I watched her through my tears. I should have taken the right hand side of the road all the way up to the crosswalk and then allowed the school patrol to escort me to the other side of the street.

OK, I thought, I've got it now.

I tried it the next day, hoping that the school patrol wouldn't show up in the class. Boy, was I was happy when they didn't appear!

As a third grader I was waiting in line for lunch, when the biggest boy in the class gave everybody a "cut" ahead of me. Why? What had I done to hurt him? Why did the others take such delight in cutting in front of me? Had I offended them somehow? Or did I miss something he had said to me? As it turned out he had given everyone a password, but I didn't know the word because I never heard it.

Again, in third grade, I had to walk back home to get my Halloween costume to wear in the afternoon school parade. I had not heard the announcement the day before that we were supposed to bring our costumes to school the next morning.

When I got back to school that afternoon, I didn't know whether to put the mask on or not. I decided to put it on.

Then some kids looked at me and started saying things I couldn't understand. I could see only a small part of their faces and the hood prevented me from hearing them clearly. I was terrified.

Then other kids started talking. What were they saying? Why were they laughing at me? Now they seemed to be yelling at me. I still didn't understand. What was wrong? Didn't they like me anymore?

I turned and ran home. I wanted to be in a hole, away from everybody where I couldn't be hurt. When I was alone, I didn't have the agony of not understanding what other people were saying to me. When I was by myself, there was no one to make a fool of me.

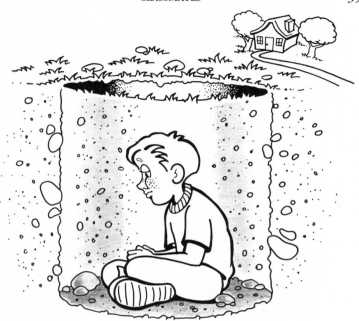

Another time, I was sitting in the classroom, and I looked up when I heard my name spoken. Obviously, the classmate who was speaking, wanted me to know that she was talking about me because she said my name loud enough for me to hear it. Four classmates looked around at her, and then at me. They were looking for some kind of appropriate response.

I was in a panic, but knew I couldn't show it. I had no idea what she had said. Her look suggested disdain, so I was darned if I was going to give her the pleasure of asking her to repeat her remarks.

I decided to shrug my shoulders and go back to doing my school work. Hopefully that was cool enough for my other classmates. I wished I could have responded to her, but I hadn't heard what she'd said.

For people with normal hearing, the sound from a noise source will enter that ear which is closest to the sound, a fraction of a second before it enters the other ear. This enables the listener to tell which direction the noise is coming from. This is called localization.

If a person loses the hearing in one ear, the ability to localize a sound source is lost. It is almost impossible to tell which direction a noise is coming from. This can result in some amusing situations for a person with a single good ear.

For instance, you are out on the playing field with your classmates and you hear your name called. You look around to see who is calling you. You don't see anybody. Then you hear your name again, louder this time. Again you look around, more intensely, but with no success.

Frustration begins to mount. You are beginning to look like a fool, and you really don't like to look dumb in front of your friends. This situation has got to be resolved, and resolved quickly!

Finally, your friend approaches you, and you spot him. Thank heavens he is laughing, saying, "I'm over here!" You smile a silly smile back, explaining to him you couldn't find him in the midst of all the other kids. Only you know this is a little white lie: you wouldn't have been able to tell where he was calling from if he was the only other kid on the whole playground!

Frequently at this age, the hard of hearing child will learn new words but be unable to pronounce them correctly. It takes practice and feedback from listeners to perfect pronunciation. Most of these mispronunciations are benign, and even children with normal hearing go through some of this.

In fifth grade I was madly in love with a girl named Sarah. I dreamed of giving her my jacket on a cold winter's night after the movies. I wanted her to think I was Prince Charming and Albert Einstein in one complete fifth grade package.

One day we were talking about women's make-up. I said something about "lickstip." She looked at me with a funny expression on her face.

"What did you say?"

"I said, 'lickstip'," I replied.

She suddenly starting laughing uncontrollably.

Oh, no! What had I done wrong now?

She said, "Oh, you mean lipstick!"

She laughed in a friendly way. Whew! She was laughing at the mispronunciation, not at me personally. I, too, joined in the laughter. Now I knew how to pronounce the word, but I had felt real anxiety there for a while.

In sixth grade I was drafted into the manly sport of football. I was in a new school and as skinny as a twig. I really didn't understand how I had gotten myself into this activity.

During our huddles, the quarterback would utter some words that were incomprehensible to me. With all the other boys around me, there was no way I was going to ask him to repeat what he had said. His helmet prevented me from watching his lips, and my helmet wasn't helping me hear.

I played right guard and I got mowed over every time. I didn't understand one play from the next. This was not my idea of fun.

THE JUNIOR HIGH
AND HIGH SCHOOL YEARS

Adolescence - A General Discussion

We all know what adolescence is about: change.

Children at this stage are beautiful to those of us who are no longer as young. They have youth - no wrinkles, no spare tire, plenty of stamina, and a full set of teeth.

But most teenagers don't feel beautiful. Their bodies are changing and change increases stress, especially when there is no control over the timing or the direction.

When I was twelve, nobody asked me, "OK, Tom, are you ready for some changes? Are you ready for a change from the body you have known for the last twelve years? Are you ready to have your voice get deeper, to grow hair under your arms, on your legs, and on your face? Are you ready to quickly become tall and skinny and have a protruding Adam's Apple? Are you ready for PIMPLES? Are you ready to feel lonely, to feel that the family that once fulfilled your emotional needs no longer does? Are you ready for the hurt of a broken relationship with someone whom you thought could fill that loneliness?"

Parents need to understand and accept the fact that the family unit alone is no longer able to fill the emotional needs of the adolescent. They still may fill part of it, but not all of it.

No matter how many worms the mother bird brings back to the nest, the fledgling isn't satisfied. It really has nothing to do with the mother bird herself. Nor is it a reflection on the mother bird as a parent. Nature simply changes the internal makeup of the adolescent so that she is no longer comfortable in the nest.

A new pair of ski boots from Mom and Dad is nice, but it does not really address the changes going on inside. It is time to start that long, lonely, and frequently painful trek toward finding a suitable mate. That is how new families are made.

So when your acts of thoughtfulness are rewarded with indifference or insolence from your teenager, don't take it personally. Your teenager isn't too happy either, and is frustrated that the parents are no longer able to fill the emotional needs as they once did.

All of the crazy fads and fashions that adolescents follow is a cry for attention: will someone other than my parents please pay attention to me?

Nature changes girls in particular, physically advertising that they are ready to leave the nest. Many thirteen year old girls seem to think they should highlight these changes with short skirts, tight pants, and make-up. This is not really a plea for sex, it's a plea for attention to fill an emotional void. My heart goes out to parents and teenagers at this stage. Making new nests and shaping adult personalities is tough on everyone.

If someone would have asked any of us if we were ready to take this trip, I'm sure many people would have said no. I think that is one reason we are not asked: we're just thrown into the sea of change with no chance to reject or change the situation.

Most of us want to get through this as rapidly as possible. Do you know many teenagers that would elect to stay fifteen? At this phase, a person is no longer a cute child, forgiven for many of his ignorant actions. He is accountable for his misjudgments. But he is not yet an adult and, therefore, is not really encouraged to do those things he feels are correct. It is a bewildering time.

Everyone would like to have as few hassles as possible going through this stage. This is a normal wish at any stage in one's life, but especially so during the teenage years.

Teenagers can not retreat into childhood to cope with their problems. Yet they do not always have the range of possibilities that adults have to tackle what is bothering them. When things go wrong, parents do not immediately come to the rescue as they may have for younger children. They expect teenagers to handle things in a more adult fashion, on their own.

Appearances can be so deceiving: I now have some small hairs on my chin, but inside I am a lot closer to twelve than to twenty. There is a lot about life that still scares me.

I still want hugs from my Dad and Mom. I might not run up to them as I did in the past, but physical contact is still very important.

When I was younger, I could put an arm around my classmates as we walked to the candy store. Now I can't do that: I would get teased for being too close to another boy.

I used to run and wrestle with the girls at school, but not anymore. You can't win. American society demands physical distance from everyone just when people need the reassurance of touch the most.

Many parents put emotional as well as physical distance between themselves and their children when their children reach adolescence. Junior is expected to be a man now, so Dad toughens up his act. No more fatherly hugs or quiet talks. Mom also has to be careful of not showing too much affection. She doesn't want her son to become dependent on her. He needs to make it as a man, to be tough. Discussions become more distant.

When I was in sixth grade, I remember having an earnest discussion with my mom in the family car at a drive-in. It was an intense conversation. I was not aware anything or anybody around us.

Suddenly the discussion was shattered by a jeering remark a boy made as he rode his bicycle by our car. Being hard of hearing, I didn't hear the full remark, and my mom told me not to pay any attention to him.

But suddenly I was aware that I was no longer just my mother's son; I was no longer just a cute little boy. I felt I had to try to make my own decision. Should I ignore the boy or not? I had to step away from my mom and decide for myself.

Never again would I have the innocent childhood talks with my mom. Adolescence had arrived. It was at that moment that I first consciously experienced the pain of being on my own, and being alone with my decisions.

There is a tremendous awakening of consciousness during these years. The individual now becomes aware that he is truly an independent soul. For the first time, he experiments with stepping outside himself and trying to see how others view him. Sometimes the view is pleasing, and other times it is not.

There are times when a person's perceived view of himself is completely wrong, but he doesn't know that. He feels he is making a correct assessment at the time. That is why it is very important for an adolescent to have some good friends he can trust. Without friends to talk and share thoughts with, the teenage years can be very lonely and frightening.

If a teenager's self-image is good before he enters adolescence, he should get through these years reasonably well. If not, then things can rapidly become sticky as the boy or girl turns to less than healthy activities. Casual sex, alcohol, drugs, and even suicide are all ways of coping with feelings of loneliness and helplessness.

The Hearing Impaired Adolescent

The hard of hearing child also wants as few problems during adolescence as possible, but he has a few additional considerations to contend with. He begins to realize the extent of his loss. The awareness that he is not functioning with the same range of abilities that his hearing peers have, can either be taken in stride or can be the basis of real withdrawal. Frequently, there is a mixture of these two.

If the hearing handicap existed during the early years of a child's life, then most likely it will be taken in stride. The parents and the child have had years to get used to the situation, so there will be a reservoir of communication between them. Problems will still occur, but the experiences and triumphs of the past will help.

If the hearing loss occurred after the age of ten, then there could be some real difficulties. Not only does the child have to cope with adolescence, but he is also dealing with something new and frightening: not being able to communicate with his parents or peers in a normal fashion. This can be devastating. Compounding the problems of withdrawal of emotional and physical support is this new communication barrier. Add to this the loneliness of these years, the longing for company outside the family circle, and you have a challenging situation.

I have known hard of hearing and deaf students, who used sign language in school without any problems. But when adolescence hit, they withdrew into themselves to the point where they didn't want to be seen in restaurants signing to their comrades. They felt that the hearing population believed they were dumb, and their fragile egos couldn't handle the idea that anyone might think that about them.

I have also had other students take things in stride during adolescence. They knew they were different in their method of communication but that didn't bother them. They actually liked being different from everybody else.

Since I was deaf in my right ear from an early age, I had time to get used to dealing with my deafness before adolescence. I had learned to ask people to repeat what they said. "Say that again, please!" became an often used phrase. I found it helped to walk on the right side of people so that my good ear was closest to them. I had also learned where to sit at restaurants so that the noise in the room was kept to a minimum. I knew I should sit in the front of the classroom, and not be shy about asking the teacher to repeat a remark. I had coped reasonably well as far as I was concerned.

Then suddenly at the age of twelve, life became a lot more difficult. My left inner ear would periodically accumulate too much fluid. It would happen without warning, and then I could hardly hear anything. I would go to bed at night and wake up the next morning functionally deaf. I can assure you, that at the age of twelve, I didn't like it one bit. I was scared. I suddenly had a whole new hearing disability to adjust to - in addition to adjusting to adolescence!

These trips into the world of the deaf usually lasted for two weeks, sometimes longer. One lasted for three years. Although I have not had a recurrence of this particular deafness for over fifteen years, those experiences made a lasting impression on me: I appreciate the music I hear every day.

Before this type of deafness occurred, my family was used to contending with a hard of hearing child whose loss was in just one ear. They didn't have to adjust too much to deal with that handicap. Consequently, none of us knew how to deal with this new situation. I felt totally cut off from everybody: I knew no deaf people and I had never seen sign language.

I vividly remember waking up one morning at my cousin's house and not being able to hear a thing: during the night my ear had become plugged. I was awake before my cousins so I had plenty of time to panic. I had no escape. Soon they were going to wake up and start talking to me. What was I going to say to them?

One of my cousins woke up and said something. I mumbled "Hmm", and walked out of the room in total fear. He must have thought that I was a complete idiot.

I met my mom and her sister in another part of the house, and they said something to me. I thought it was, "Good morning, Tom."

I hoped so and said, "Good morning," in return.

Then I fled out of the house so I could be alone.

Again, I wanted to crawl into a hole, where there was nobody to communicate with, somewhere I would not look like a fool or have to struggle to respond to somebody talking to me.

My mom took me to an ear clinic. The doctors diagnosed the problem as a form of Meniere's Disease. They didn't know what caused it, but they did know the effect: too much fluid in the inner ear resulted in a hearing loss. Sometimes this loss was temporary, and at other times it could be permanent. The hearing that remained was frequently distorted, and recruitment (sensitivity to loud noises) made things even more difficult.

All I knew was that this was no fun, nobody could really do anything about it, and I had to live with it.

The doctor suggested the use of a hearing aid when my ear became plugged, so we went to a hearing aid store.

I didn't like the idea of being different, and I disliked like the idea of something that would advertise my differences even more. That hearing aid was the equivalent of a billboard. Wearing glasses for the first time in school was bad enough. Being called "four-eyes" by some so-called friends was a part of the pain of dealing with schoolmates. But not even my real friends had ever seen a hearing aid before. This *was* different.

I remember the hearing aid salesman admonishing me to make sure I used the hearing aid everyday. Being young and brash, I asked him what would happen if I decided not to use his little device. He told me that I would lose the ability to pronounce words properly.

Oh great! Not only would I not be able to hear others, but I would also lose my ability to speak clearly. Although it is generally true that the more profound the hearing loss, the greater the speech impairment (since the speaker can not monitor how his speech sounds), this varies greatly among individuals over a wide range of hearing losses. A person who loses his hearing at the age of three months is obviously going to feel the effects of such a loss much more than an adult who has already developed speech. The adult will suffer some impairment, but it is highly doubtful that she will lose the ability to speak understandably.

I didn't think I would suffer such a calamity. I felt the hearing aid salesman was wrong. I knew myself. After he made that statement, I discounted every thing else he said to me. Of course, I didn't say that to him. I didn't tell my mother what I thought either. She had done the best she could to help me. There was no way I was going to criticize her efforts, even if I did think this man was a little bit off.

Hard of hearing children, and particularly deaf children, receive all kinds of advice from many sources. It is usually filtered by the child to see if it fits and feels right. Most of this advice is given by hearing individuals who frequently do not understand the entire problem. They understand the outward signs, symptoms, and generally accepted courses of action for a particular problem, but the child is the one who experiences the hidden problems of the handicap. Through no fault of his own the hearing person just doesn't completely comprehend. So deaf children learn early to use their own judgement. This frustrates many hearing teachers who deal with deaf and hard of hearing students.

I tried to make light of my hearing aid in front of my contemporaries. One way to do that was to make up stories about all the conversations I could eavesdrop on. I told my friends they couldn't hear these stories because they didn't have hearing aids. I knew they couldn't possibly correct my recounting of these conversations because the conversations didn't exist.

Because my left ear stopped up only periodically, I was able to attend regular schools. There was a tremendous amount of anxiety on my part though, because I was unable to predict whether or not I was going to be able to hear from one day to the next. There were many days when I would miss a lot of the classroom conversation. I was, however, able to get the main idea, and my grades stayed above average.

When I was in eighth grade, I even convinced my parents to allow me to attend my father's prep school, Culver Military Academy. Academically, this was the best thing that could have happened to me. This school was top notch and the teachers were exceptional. It was a good thing, though, that I was so ignorant of the difficulties I was to encounter. I doubt very much that I would have elected such a route if I had known what was coming. Being ignorant of these challenges, I coped with them as they came and am pleased to have attended this outstanding school.

For the amusement of some readers and to give readers some understanding of the situations the hard of hearing have to face, I would like to relate several incidents that occurred during my four years at Culver.

Registration day came. There I was, a freshman, only fourteen years old. My thoughts ran something like this:

This campus is big! How am I ever going to learn how to get around this place?

And look how big and tough looking those senior officers are! They are wearing uniforms and carrying sabers. They know about everything here. I know nothing.

And that's the easy part. The night before, my good ear plugged up and now I can't hear a damn thing. What a great way for things to start out!

My mother brought me here to Indiana all the way from California. But I have to be tough in front of all the other cadets; there is no way I am going to tell her how lost I am.

I shake her hand, saying, "Good-bye, Mom. Thanks for bringing me here."

I turn to go into the barracks. OK kid, now you are really on your own. I guess it won't take long for people to think I am pretty dumb when I don't respond to what they are saying, or even worse, when I respond inappropriately.

Just because a person is deaf does not mean he is stupid. I can recall many of my deaf students who were much more capable than I was in mathematics. But if you put those students and me, in a situation where it is necessary to hear to solve a problem, then I would appear much more intelligent. Appearances can be deceiving. In any case, let's go back to Culver and adolescence, where appearances seemed to be reality.

6:30 a.m. Reveille. Time to face my first day in a military environment without much hearing.

What woke me up? I didn't hear the bell in the hallway. Nor did I hear the cannon boom across the lake. I felt the vibrations coming from the floor as my roommate walked around in our room. I opened my eyes. He had already made his bed. Gosh, I'd better get going.

Out of desperation, I put on my hearing aid. The billboard goes up, I have no choice: some noise is better than no noise; some words getting through are better than no words. It is a great effort. The noise is louder, but understanding the words is still an iffy proposition.

The "battery" (a group of about sixty boys in an artillery unit) is out drilling. We are learning how to march. Different commands mean different movements.

"Right turn!" means each cadet in the front line of a marching column of cadets turns to his right. The succeeding lines of cadets continue marching forward until they reach the same point and then they, too, make an abrupt right turn. From a distance it looks something like a snake making a sharp right turn.

"Right flank!", means the entire column immediately turns to the right, all at the same time. It is a vastly different maneuver.

Needless to say, if the command given is "Right flank!" rather than "Right turn!" and some cadet continues to walk straight ahead, he will mess up the entire unit. And nobody likes an oaf who messes up everybody else's efforts.

The proper sequence of orders is "Right flank!", followed by a pause for the right step and then "March!" At the command "March!" the action commences.

Well, I hear the words "Right mnvcke!" Panic! Which one is it? At the next command, "March!", do I walk straight or turn to the right? I blow it repeatedly. Are the officers happy with me? Are the other cadets happy with me?

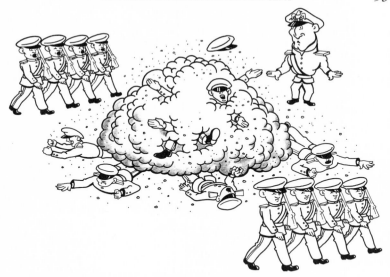

I soon become good at responding very quickly: I watch the other cadets intensely. I follow their movements instantly and am able to get by. I'm learning.

While I am out on the drill field, the hearing aid has helped some. But remember the wind noise? It was there. And the commander was considerably farther than five feet away from me when he was barking out his orders. Of course when I messed up, he and the other officers obligingly reduced that distance to inches!

One additional thought about hearing aids and high school students. No one is going to make things more difficult for themselves than they have to. When there is an easier way to do things, that is the way people will do them. This includes using hearing aids: if the benefits of easier communication outweigh the frustrations and limitations of these devices, then a person is going to use them; if not, then the aid will not be used. The only person who knows whether the device is actually providing benefit is the person who wears the aid, not the person selling the aid, not the person fitting the aid, not the teacher of the deaf, and not the parent. This is particularly true by the time a person is in high school. If a person is old enough to drive a car, then he is old enough to decide whether a hearing aid is making life easier or not.

While I was teaching, I remember other high school teachers who would frequently demand that all the students use their hearing aids. These teachers had normal hearing. My hearing fluctuated, so I wore my hearing aid at some times but not at others. This proved to be confusing to some teachers. They wanted to recruit me into setting an example for the students. I tried to explain that there are good days and there are bad days, at least in my case, when it came to using the aid.

As a result of my own experience, I strongly urge parents to let their teenagers decide for themselves whether their aid will help or not. Kids are not stupid. No student that I have known, purposely made communication more difficult. Because each hearing loss is unique, only the person involved can tell if an aid is helping.

Getting back to Culver, at every formation or formal grouping of cadets, there is a roll call, in which the names of the cadets are called out, one by one, by the first sergeant. The cadet is expected to come to attention after his name is called, respond by saying loudly, "Here, sir!", and then return to a parade rest stance.

Now imagine that a name is called out but you can't hear what it is. You come to attention and yell out, "Here, sir!" But it is not your name. The other cadets and officers are going to quickly become convinced that you are loony. Or what if your name is called out, and you don't respond? Did you skip out of the required formation? That is punishable by marching extra-duty hours.

Could it be that you just are not paying attention? That makes more work for the first sergeant, since he has to repeat your name and that holds up the entire battery. They want to be done with it, so they can go and get something to eat.

You hear the first sergeant call out a name. Was that your name? Should you respond? You look at him intensely. You are supposed to look straight ahead, so you look out of the corner of your eye. If you don't think you heard another cadet respond and you see the first sergeant begin to raise his face from the roster, you immediately respond a belated, "Here, sir!" He goes on with the list of names, thank God. You held things up but not by too much.

Later, I learned to check the roster before the time of assembly. I would count the number of names. I would then know when to expect my name to be called. This method worked ninety-five percent of the time. The other five percent of the time I'm sure I looked like a fool, but this only happened once in a great while.

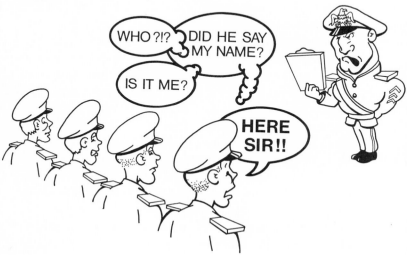

Eventually I became a senior endowed with rank and a knowledge of what was going on. This was fine, but frustrating situations still developed. The difficulty of hearing the commands was no different for me as a senior than as a freshman.

I can remember when I was an acting lieutenant in charge of thirty cadets in the first platoon. The battery commander would yell out a marching order to the whole battery. It was the responsibility of the two platoon commanders to repeat this command to each of our platoons. After that, at the precise moment he wanted the marching order executed, the battery commander would yell, "March!"

We are marching along and the commander yells out, "Right megytr!"

Oh great! I've got to repeat that to the thirty cadets under my command. They heard it, but I didn't.

I yell out, "Right megytr!"

If I am worried about not even getting close to what the commander has said, I make a point of looking sharply to the right or left as I mumble the order. That makes it look as though something had severely distracted my attention and prevented me from repeating the command in a precise manner.

I am praying that everybody in my platoon heard the correct command from the commander. Then they would know what to do, even though their platoon leader mumbled the orders.

I hear the commander yell, "March!" I watch what happens. Thank heavens everybody heard the battery commander's initial order and are moving as they are supposed to. Whew!

This happened repeatedly, and I was lucky most of the time.

I wonder, in retrospect, how many of my fellow cadets knew that I was acting, that inside I was constantly in fear of making a total fool out of myself. Rank would not protect me from ridicule.

In a boys military school, weakness, even the perception of weakness, is immediately noticed. Compassion for others is a virtue learned over time, a sign of maturity. Most high school boys are still too young to exhibit this trait. Toughness is the order of the day. The idea of going up to my fellow cadets and calmly explaining my problem to them, was unthinkable. The idea appeals to an adult, but as an adolescent dealing with other adolescents on a daily basis, especially in a military school, I knew there was just no way that kind of conversation could happen. Adults have to understand that it is not very easy to calmly inform your classmates that you are different. Being different carried the chance of not being accepted. No way.

If you are different by choice, that is one thing. You have control over your decision; you elected not to be a part of a group. But if the choice is not yours, if you are different due to circumstances beyond your control, then there is a sense of helplessness. This is doubly frustrating if you feel you can't do anything about it.

The hard of hearing or deaf person finds it very difficult to fit into a hearing group because he can not keep up with the antics and conversation of the group. He can't defend himself when the group's ridicule focuses on him, because he doesn't understand precisely what the jokes are. It's a tough time at any age.

THE ADULT YEARS

College

In many people's opinion the college years are the best years. I will not argue with that. Life is still full of promise for the future. You're young, but old enough to be given most of the respect adults have. There are no bills, no spouse, and no children. Since you probably don't have a full time job, you have time to enjoy life. You do have one thing to concern yourself with, getting grades good enough to justify your otherwise abundant free time.

I was successful in college. My undergraduate studies were in business administration at Babson College in Wellesley, Massachusetts. I was on the dean's list repeatedly and graduated with honors. My master's degree was also in business administration and this also was earned with honors.

Later, I went to the University of Northern Colorado in Greeley, Colorado, to earn a master's degree in special education with the acoustically handicapped. My grades were above average.

The point here is not to impress anyone, but to show that I was able to successfully meet the challenges of the normal college classroom. I had learned good study habits and discipline from my Culver experience. In college, as a hard of hearing student I had to learn a few additional tricks to help me through. It was generally not hard but took some imagination to find ways to master various situations.

If you are enrolled in a class that has two hundred students, you had better make sure you get into the classroom early so you can grab one of the front seats. If you are late and end up in the back of the classroom you won't be able to hear the lecture.

In addition, in your larger classes it is difficult to overcome a sense of guilt of using everyone else's time when you want to ask the professor a question. This is hard enough for a regular student. The hard of hearing person is probably not going to assert himself by asking a question on a matter that he thinks everybody else understands.

Even in moderately large classes of forty-five students, it is very difficult for the hard of hearing person to follow classroom conversations. The classroom is larger and the distance between you, the other students, and the teacher are much greater. The sound sources are farther away.

I can remember several times wanting very badly to participate in classroom discussions. The teacher had just made a few comments on a certain point. She then called upon another student in the class who wanted to make a point or ask a question. The student made some comments that I could not understand. Nevertheless, after he finished talking, I raised my hand to add what I thought was important.

Sometimes the thrust of my message was almost exactly what the first student had said. The expression on the teacher's face told me that.

At other times the point I was trying to make really didn't have a thing to do with the current topic. The look on the teacher's face was a little different, but it also told me that I had blown it.

Then there were the times when a student decided to directly question some of the points I was presenting to the class. If I couldn't hear the point or specific rebuttal being voiced, it was very difficult to participate in the debate in an intelligent fashion.

So I quickly learned to keep my mouth shut in the larger classrooms. I sometimes thought I could add to the discussion, but it didn't seem to be worth the risk of getting disdainful looks. It was just easier not to bother the teacher or the class.

One of the graces of being a college student is that the system treats you with a little more dignity than when you are in fifth grade. You are able to structure your class schedule and raise points of discussion with your teachers.

A rather pleasant by-product of this for me was the opportunity to openly copy notes from my fellow classmates during lectures. When I was not able to hear what the teacher was saying, I would look around the classroom for a student who seemed to be a good note taker. I would then make it a point of sitting next to this person and ask for his permission to look at his notes during the lecture. I could then follow the lecture and copy the notes.

Later, during my studies for my masters in special education, I met other students who had a much greater hearing loss than mine. They had taken this note taking system one step further: they would ask a note taker to place a piece of carbon paper underneath his own notebook sheet. At the end of the class, the note taker would then simply give the carbon copy to the hearing impaired student.

This worked very well, particularly for those students who were completely deaf. They were then able to focus on a signing interpreter who would be standing next to the lecturer. They could watch what was being said and still have a copy of the lecture in note form.

Youth is a time to try things that older and wiser people would hesitate to do. When I was younger I did some things that I might balk at today. I took up flying and earned my commercial, instrument, multi-engine, and flight instructor ratings. My father was a pilot, so in spite of my hearing loss, I didn't see why I couldn't become one, too. It was a lot of work, but also a lot of fun.

My hearing problem was overcome by patient flight instructors and by using earphones. With these wonderful devices the voice of the control tower or "center" was right inside my ear, clear, crisp, and a volume that I could set at my discretion.

In addition, the headphones blocked out engine and wind noises that could have made communication more difficult for me. The FAA, to their credit, wanted to make sure I was actually able to communicate with their ground controllers, so I went up for a special test with one of their examiners. I won their approval and have been enjoying flying for the last twenty years without any problems. I even flew a DC-3 for an oil company in Alaska during the summer of '69.

I also took up scuba diving and sport parachuting. These are fun but not without danger. One has to understand what is necessary for safety; a misunderstanding can be fatal. But if an individual exercises attention and has patient instructors, it can be done.

I am trying to show that one should not be too quick to presume limitations for hard of hearing or deaf people. With enough desire, patience, and time, almost anything is within their grasp.

Motivation, self-esteem, parental support, teacher support, intelligence, and environment all play a part. I believe that if an individual is not prepared for defeat by well meaning advice, that he will frequently accomplish a lot more than many people believed possible. That is why I caution parents and teachers to be very careful in setting limits on the dreams of their children or pupils. If the dreams are truly unrealistic, the children will find that out for themselves. Give them the freedom to pursue their dreams. They might just beat the odds.

I am not suggesting that anything is possible. That sounds nice, but reality will dictate some limits. Each individual will accomplish things in a manner and to a degree to which he is most comfortable. The degree of hearing loss is only one factor.

If my parents had any reservations about my ability to become a pilot, a scuba diver, a parachutist, or anything else that I have tried so far, they kept me in the dark about them. That suits me just fine.

I do believe that if they had expressed doubts as to my ability to accomplish any of these things, I might have given up. There were times when my hearing did make it tough. But nobody told me it was too tough, so I kept plugging away.

Before leaving the college years, I want to relate another interesting experience. I had returned to college at the University of Northern Colorado to get a degree in teaching the hearing impaired. I was just learning sign language and wanted to practice it with everyone I ran into both on and off campus.

I heard there was a conference of deaf educators meeting in Denver one weekend, so I decided to go down to meet some people in my newly chosen profession. Of course, I wanted to show them that I was making a sincere effort to learn and use sign language, so I signed during every conversation. I thought I was doing a pretty good job. I noticed that I kept getting strange looks from several people. I didn't understand why, but I figured that maybe I was making an occasional mistake.

After a while, I was taken aside by one of my colleagues from the college. He told me this was a conference of educators that felt very strongly that the deaf should not be taught the use of sign language! The rationale was, that it is a hearing world and the hearing population is not going to learn to use signs just for the benefit of the deaf population. So the deaf need to learn to cope without signs. No wonder I had received those looks. Boy, was I ignorant of the divergent opinions in this field!

At the time, my hearing in my good ear was down, so I was functioning pretty much at the deaf level. I asked my friend exactly how was I supposed to understand the coming lecture in the auditorium when I was sitting at the back of this large group of people.

"Well, Tom, don't you know?" he said, smiling politely. "You are just supposed to make the most of your residual hearing."

I didn't pour my Coke directly on his tie because I understood from his smile that he, too, thought the whole thing was preposterous.

Because I was an adult, I was polite for the rest of the conference. I didn't tell the people there that I sat through the major address of their conference without understanding a single word. I didn't tell them that I was very thankful that as a child I had been able to hear enough to get by in a normal classroom. Thankful I was not deaf and subjected to their idea of breaking down communication barriers by "using the most of my residual hearing."

I do know some deaf students who have succeeded without the use of signs, but there are very few. What happens to those who don't succeed? At what time and at what age can anyone determine whether the use of sign language would be better? How much communication and time for language development has been lost at this point? Enough said.

Work

Let's face it, the phone bill has to be paid. Your parents were nice enough to cover your use of the telephone for the first eighteen years of your life, but eventually you get the joy of assuming the responsibilities of an adult. One of those responsibilities is paying the bills. Inspiring you to reach for the stars is one thing. Living from day to day with the kind of job you're going to do is another.

What kind of job do you want? Do you want a job that deals with people or with machines? A job that is outdoors or indoors? A noisy environment or a quiet one? Do you like to work with figures or with words? Do you thrive on meeting the challenges of deadlines? Do you want to be intellectually challenged or just told what to do? What kind of people do you want to associate with? The questions go on and on.

Successfully answering them requires soul searching. From day to day, exactly what do you want to do? Not what does your mom want you to do, or your dad, or your sister or brother, but what exactly do you want to do?

The hard of hearing or deaf person has to temper his desires with reality. Like everybody else he has to pay the bills, but the kinds of jobs that are feasible for him are somewhat fewer than those available for hearing people. In the real world the hard of hearing or deaf person is going to have to deal with people who really don't care about his problems.

Employers and co-workers have enough personal problems of their own. They also have to contend with normal business problems: deadlines, quotas, personnel management headaches, past due accounts, and so on. If these problems are not dealt with, then the worker himself may become vulnerable. His job, and the time he must devote to insuring its continuity, will take precedence over someone else's hearing problems.

The hard of hearing person and especially the deaf person, has to look for a job that he can comfortably and successfully perform day in and day out on his own.

A sales job communicating with many hearing individuals would probably be highly stressful for anyone with impaired hearing. Dealing with large groups would also be a problem; it is difficult for people with a hearing loss to hear people speaking from the back of a large room.

I taught mathematics to deaf students for seven years. The class size was never more than twelve. Being in front of this group did not bother me at all because our communication involved the constant use of sign language. If a student wanted to ask me a question he would sign to me. If my hearing was not up to par that day it posed no real problems, I could just watch the student's signs.

Recently I moved to a small town in Idaho. McCall is too small to have a program for the deaf, but I wanted to stay in touch with high school students and continue teaching algebra. I decided to experiment by substitute teaching for a day at the high school.

Now, everybody knows that the substitute is fair game. The sub really doesn't know what is going on, and both the kids and the sub know that. Things can quickly become very interesting.

My experience subbing in the high school couldn't have been better. The students were courteous, helpful, and did not take advantage of me. The problem was my hearing. Instead of having ten students, I was now confronted with thirty. When a student in the back of the class said something it was as though he was a mile away. I had to strain to hear the entire day. I got by, but it was more of an effort to me than it was worth. So much for subbing in a normal classroom.

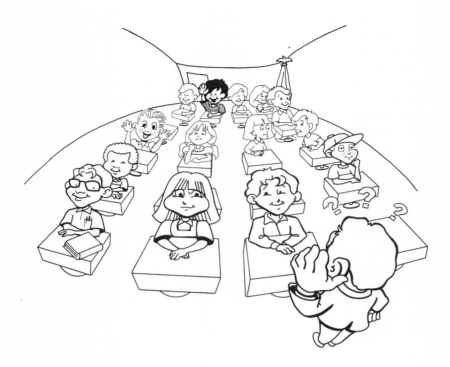

I decided to try tutoring. During an intense hour, I could frequently clear up a student's frustration with algebra. This restored his confidence and smiles, and brought me no end of satisfaction and personal joy. The urge to teach was fulfilled and my limited hearing didn't get in the way.

I am trying to show that there are ways to blend interests, ability, and reality when searching for a job.

With that said, it must be noted that it was possible for Ronald Reagan, who is hard of hearing, to become president.

I have great respect for the man who frequently succeeded in addressing a hostile press corps during his news conferences. Dealing with groups is especially tough for the hard of hearing. Add to that several factors: he was using a hearing aid, the meetings were held in a large room, he was confronted by a very large group of people, and many of these people were shouting at him at the same time. With all of that to hinder the president from receiving a full question from a single voice, it is a wonder he didn't misunderstand all of the questions thrown at him. I also understand why he might not have wanted to ask a reporter to repeat a question. Saying "Say that again, please!" too many times could have made him look like a fool.

So what do you do? You keep smiling, nod your head, and hopefully they won't know how much you've missed. You're not dumb or senile, but you are having a devil of a time hearing. I am not sure Mr. Reagan did this, but I would not be surprised, given the nature of hearing impairment.

Yes, your hard of hearing child could become president, but as I said before, some jobs are easier than others. Your child will know how he wants to go through life. There will be some trials, some false starts, but he will eventually make it in his own way.

Later Years

I must admit, this part of the book involves more speculation than actual experience. I can relate to the reader, though, my feelings in regards to some situations I have encountered as an older uncle.

The central problem of hearing loss is the diminished capacity to communicate with one's fellow human beings. This is frustrating enough when it is a problem in and of itself, but when other problems of the aging process are added, it can be even more distressing.

When a person is approaching retirement small doubts start creeping in. What will I be good for after I stop working here? What will happen to my standard of living on my retirement income? What will I do with all my free time?

Then there are the physical aspects of growing older. The body is just not the same. The eyes don't focus as quickly, the legs don't bend as readily, the back is not as flexible, the teeth are not as secure as they once were, and the hearing is not as keen as it once was.

This aging process is part of life. Its effects do not mean you are less of a person. Indeed, wisdom, the compassion for understanding life, and an ability to see true beauty in people and nature often come only with the passage of time. Youth often has beauty on the surface, but rarely wisdom inside. Some people accept this without too much fuss. They may exercise to keep themselves in shape, but do not resist this natural process of life. I believe this is called "aging gracefully."

Others do everything to stop the aging process, and are continuously frustrated and fearful about something they can not control. Life becomes an endless blur of new miracle diets, exercise programs, and face lifts.

If in addition to all the other problems of aging, a person suffers the loss of being able to communicate with friends, then he may easily feel worth even less.

One great fear of older people is losing contact with loved ones. Becoming senile or being considered senile by others, especially loved ones, is a very frightening thought. The behavior pattern of the hard of hearing has many of the same outward symptoms as senility. You miss many of the jokes at parties. You don't understand what your spouse is trying to say to you. You can't seem to follow spoken directions. People confuse you. You withdraw out of fear and seek solitude even from your spouse to avoid being embarrassed or embarrassing someone you love.

If you are becoming hard of hearing you have got to let your friends know. Ask them to speak a little louder. True friends will have no problem with this. They will want to do what they can for you, but again, you have to let them know. It is only fair to them, and it will make your life a whole lot easier.

Explore using a hearing aid. They have helped a great many people. If an older relative of yours is resisting the use of a hearing aid, have patience. Adjustments take time.

Hearing spouses and friends must realize that hearing aids help sometimes, but they do not restore hearing. Only if the benefits of the aid overwhelm the inherent limitations will a person elect to wear it. Anything short of this will be met with resistance.

I understand the frustration of not being able to freely communicate with younger relatives. I have a nephew and a niece, ages seven and nine. Their voices in the upper frequency range are difficult for me to hear. In addition they speak quietly, since they are shy when addressing an adult.

I really want to give them all the attention I can, play with them, build log cabins, give them bear hugs, etc. But I have a hearing problem. I don't want to make my niece or nephew feel that they have to make any special efforts to communicate with me. I don't want to put them out.

When they say something to me I frequently have to ask them to say it twice, and sometimes a third time. The children squirm as though they are being put on the witness stand. I hate doing that to them.

One solution is for me to stay away from the children, keeping busy helping their parents with some made up chore. Then the children will not have the opportunity to enter into a conversation with me. They will not have to be asked to repeat anything, and I will have fewer chances of looking like a fool.

Extrapolate this to other, initially closer relationships, and you'll see possibilities for tragic losses. It is particularly sad when one sees this withdrawal occur between spouses. A man losses his hearing and withdraws from his wife; she does not understand and in turn withdraws. How unfortunate this is.

The best friend in such a situation is one who will stand by and make sure the hard of hearing or deaf person understands the conversation going on. It takes a lot of patience. Through time the hearing impaired person will learn that there are friends who will not ridicule him when he does not understand but show compassion and support. They will repeat sentences without allowing a look of exasperation to appear on their faces. They will ask the person who has difficulty hearing where he wants to sit at the table, to make communication easiest for him. They will include him in their discussions and make sure he understands what is being discussed. Their support and patience will show him that he does not have to withdraw; he is among friends who care about him and understand his hearing impairment.

• • • • • • • • • • • • •

CHAPTER II

TEACHERS AND PARENTS

INTRODUCTION TO CHAPTER II

This section of the book reflects the insights of a group of teachers and parents, who have shown an extraordinary sense of understanding of the world of the hard of hearing and the deaf. Some of these participants are themselves deaf, some are teachers of the deaf, some are hard of hearing, and some have normal hearing.

A variety of families are represented in the group. Some are hard of hearing parents with hearing children. Some are hearing parents who have raised deaf children. One woman has a profound hearing loss but her husband has normal hearing. Another young lady with a severe hearing loss, whose first husband was deaf, is now married to a man with normal hearing.

Some are uniquely qualified because they are members of more than one of these groups. Some are teachers of the deaf who also have deaf children. Some are teachers of the deaf and are deaf or hard of hearing themselves. A couple of the deaf participants are teachers of the deaf who have hearing children. There is broad range of perspectives here. It is hoped that readers will be able to use these interviews to avoid, or minimize many of the frustrations these people have experienced.

Some of the answers may not seem to directly answer the questions and may seem to go off on a tangent. I have elected not to break up the flow of the interviews, because they often contain important information which has more impact when left in its original context.

THE PARTICIPANTS

Joseph Livingston

Normal hearing

M.A. in audiology

Doctoral work in audiology

Teacher of the deaf and hard of hearing

School audiologist

Medical clinic audiologist

Former director of teacher training for teachers of the deaf at the University of Northern Colorado

Former director of the Aspen Camp School for the Deaf

Cheryl Deconde Johnson

Normal hearing

Daughter, Jennifer, has 75 db[1] bilateral hearing loss as a result of mother's rubella during pregnancy.

B.A. in speech pathology and audiology

M.A. in audiology

Ph.D. in special education administration

Professionally involved in audiology and deaf education since 1976.

Andrew Nielsen

Normal hearing

Deaf son, Joel

B.A. in social studies

M.A. in teaching the acoustically handicapped

Teacher for 24 years, nineteen with hearing impaired students preschool through high school, in both residential and day school settings

---

[1]"DB" referred to here means decibels. This is a unit for measuring the relative loudness of a sound.

Currently teaching middle school and high school hearing impaired students language arts and individualized mathematics programs.

Teaches hearing students sign language classes.

Coaches hearing impaired students in basketball.

Paula Smith

Profound hearing loss since the age of three due to spinal meningitis

Enrolled in the San Francisco Hearing and Speech Center for speech therapy.

Attended public elementary school in a mainstreamed program for the hard of hearing.

Attended regular junior high and high schools graduating, seventh out of a class of forty-one.

B.A. in special education from Central Washington State University, 1972

M.S. in rehabilitation counseling from University of Arizona, 1980

Taught primary hearing impaired, language deprived students in Mukilteo, Washington, for two years.

Resource teacher for the hearing impaired in Dutch Harbor, Alaska, for three years

State vocational rehabilitation counselor for the deaf in Los Angeles for four years

Currently vocational services specialist at Phoenix Day School for the Deaf

Married to a hearing man, Chuck.

Daughter, Amy born in October 1988 has normal hearing.

Chuck Smith

Husband of Paula Smith

Normal hearing

Donald Kitson

Deaf due to birth injury

Attended regular schools with the help of his mother, a teacher.

Learned sign language at nineteen at Gallaudet University.

B.A. in mathematics and physics from Gallaudet

M.Ed. in mathematics education from the University of Northern Florida

M.A. in supervisor administration in deaf education from the California State University in Northridge, 1981

Formerly married to a woman deaf since the age of three due to scarlet fever

Two sons with normal hearing

Taught physics and coached football at Gallaudet University for two years.

Taught high school mathematics and coached football and track at Florida School for the Deaf for five years.

Taught junior and senior high school deaf students at Corpus Christi, Texas, for three years.

Currently teaching and coaching all varsity sports at Phoenix Day School for the Deaf.

Ms. Linda Storch

Born profoundly deaf second of five children, four of whom were born deaf.

Mother hard of hearing, father deaf

Went to oral schools for the deaf in Chicago; wore hearing aids throughout her education.

Was not permitted to learn or use sign language in school; learned sign language from her parents.

Placed in a mainstream program in sixth grade.

Hard of hearing daughter, Amy

Ms. Yita Harrison

Became deaf during her teens as a result of spinal meningitis and five double mastoids.

Went to regular schools through high school, and attended the University of Arizona for one year.

B.A. in special education from Gallaudet College

Taught at Indiana State School for the Deaf

Taught in Phoenix Union high schools and adult education classes for the deaf for fifteen years.

Taught sign language to hearing individuals for twenty years at community colleges and universities in the Phoenix and Tempe areas.

Teacher at the Interpreters' Training Program in Phoenix

Currently teaching at Phoenix Day School for the Deaf, where she has taught for nineteen years.

Linda and Lawrence Hawbaker

Both have normal hearing.

Son, Bobby, born profoundly deaf

Helga Simpson

Normal hearing

Daughter, Jennifer, born profoundly deaf

Ms. Pamela Pflueger:

Has normal hearing

Has a brother who is profoundly deaf due to mother's rubella during pregnancy.

M.S. in deaf education

Teacher of the hearing impaired at the elementary level

Parent-infant specialist for parents of hearing impaired infants

Consultant and employment specialist for Rehabilitation Services Administration

President of Corporate Services for the Deaf, Inc., a consulting firm providing technical development, training, marketing, and promotion services for private and public service organizations.

Patricia Pittroff Swain

Hard of hearing since birth due to RH incompatibility

Left ear initially had a 75 db hearing loss, but after birth of her first child the loss became total; right ear has a 55-60 db loss.

Has worn hearing aids since three years of age.

Her first husband was deaf; her second husband has normal hearing.

Has two hearing children.

Attended both hearing schools and schools with special educational programs.

B.A. in special education, minor in business education from University of Northern Colorado

Pauline and Richard Zamecki

Both have normal hearing.

Parents of Paula, who was born deaf as a result of maternal rubella during pregnancy.

Sheila and Ronald Kidder

Both have normal hearing.

Parents of Shannon, who was diagnosed at thirteen months as being profoundly deaf.

Both professionally licensed hearing aid dispensers.

Carolyn Lefever

Hard of hearing, 80 db high frequency loss in both ears

Started to lose her hearing at 21, due to a hereditary condition.

Attended regular schools.

B.S. in deaf education from Illinois State University, 1971

M.Ed. with specialization in reading from Arizona State University, 1981

Taught for five years in hearing impaired classrooms in public schools in Illinois.

Acting director of the Teacher Training Program for the Hearing Impaired at the University of Southern Mississippi, 1986

Classroom teacher of the deaf at Phoenix Day School for the Deaf

THE INTERVIEWS

Imagine you have to inform parents that their six-month-old infant has been diagnosed hard of hearing. What would you say to them?

Joseph Livingston:

First of all let me emphasize that I am no longer a professional in this field. Though I have worked for many years in the fields of audiology and deaf education, I am no longer a practicing professional. My opinions are a result of my past experiences, and I encourage anyone who is seeking information in this field to contact those professionals who are currently working in this area on a daily basis.

In answer to your question, I strongly encourage the parents to see professionals.

I spent six years of my professional life when I was doing exactly this; checking children with hearing losses. It was my job to inform the parents of the test results and to try to provide some guidance. To do a good job you have to have a high level of empathy for the parents. You also have to have a real empathy for the children.

By professional, I mean a good otologist who probably would have an audiologist working with him. Between them they could come up with some data that would give, if not concrete answers, at least some very good indications as to what the problem is. Secondly, I recommend that if there is a hearing loss, that the parents and child visit a teacher of the deaf.

The important thing is that the parents must not hesitate to see a true professional who is active in the field, someone who is willing to spend time with the parents for counseling and guidance. Make no mistake about it, a situation such as this will require a lot of time.

In the past, when it was my position to personally inform the parents that their child had a loss, I always felt that complete honesty was the best approach. As you know when you are testing a young child, say from zero to six months, you have an impression of what his hearing is, but you can't put absolute numbers on it.

Not being able to put absolute numbers on the test result should not be a major concern at this stage. The important thing is to establish whether there is a hearing loss or not. Expressing the loss in terms of mild, moderate, or severe means more to many parents than exact, but unfamiliar measurements such as a 45 db loss or an 80 db loss.

As I said, I always felt it was much better to be as honest as I could with the parents. If I thought it was a serious loss, I would tell them. If I felt there was a hearing loss, but that I could not tell to what degree or if I felt it was a moderate loss, I would try to tell them that also.

The second thing I tried to let them know was that a problem needed to be dealt with and that it would require ongoing treatment. This kind of problem would not go away tomorrow.

Many times the parents were relieved to learn what was causing the problem. At least now they knew what they are dealing with. Confirmation by a professional gives the problem a name and permits the parents to start to minimizing its effects.

Remember that at six months or even up to eleven months, the observable everyday behavior of a deaf child is not drastically different from that of a hearing child. The first thing you start to notice is that the child does not seem to respond to you. Many parents, because they notice that their child is not responding to the environment, have fears of mental retardation.

I think one of the important things for the professional in this area is to work with the parents, to encourage them, and to help them get started on an educational program. Depending on the community where the parents are living, there may be children's hospitals and professional clinics, both public and private, where some very excellent language and speech development work is done. Most hospitals that have otology clinics will have educational or counseling systems in place. I encourage parents to seek these places out as quickly as possible. Try to get involved with a program that specializes in speech pathology for deaf education, particularly those programs that address themselves to early childhood.

Once you begin a program, stay with that program unless progress is not being made. I do not feel it is in the child's interest to jump around from program to program. The child can become so confused that he becomes lost to the educational process.

Cheryl Deconde Johnson:

Since I am a diagnostician, I am frequently in this situation. I am often the person who informs the parents. Usually the parents have been referred because a potential hearing problem is suspected.

Since the news of a hearing impairment has been anticipated for a child with a severe or profound loss, situations where parents are totally unsuspecting are infrequent. For children with a mild or moderate hearing impairment however, the diagnosis can be initially startling.

In response to how I would inform them: first of all, I would almost never make a diagnosis on the basis of one assessment. Also, I make sure that at least one parent is always present with me during the evaluation. When the parent is in the room with the child during the evaluation, he is able to see how his child is responding. I talk with the parent to explain what the child should be doing as we are conducting the evaluation. The parent can usually see the significance of his child's abnormal responses to the test stimuli by observing the testing.

Depending on the degree of impairment that I see, I may ask the parents to bring their child back in about a week to repeat the evaluation. During this week I ask the parents to do some things with their child as an informal assessment. After the second evaluation, I sit down with the parents and discuss the results and their ramifications.

At this time I may experiment with hearing aids and make ear mold impressions. I give the parents some reading material and ask them to return for follow-up testing and discussion.

A medical referral is also made. At a minimum, medical consultation must include an otologic examination. The extent of medical care and treatment depends on the nature of the hearing impairment. After medical clearance is obtained, I schedule another appointment for the purpose of fitting hearing aids on the child.

Immediately after all the assessments have been completed and the hearing aids have been fitted, the child is started on a hearing aid orientation program. At the same time I begin to explain to the parents the various philosophies of communication and education and ask them to consider the different approaches.

The Denver Ear Institute has set up a clearing-house where parents can get information and look at videos of the different types of programs and approaches used for teaching the hearing impaired. It has become a good resource for parents and strives to remain factual and unbiased in its presentations. I have found it critical for parents to know the options that are available to them. The program that will succeed is usually the one the parents feel most comfortable with.

They may want to try a program but after a year decide to change to a different one. It is during the initial period that this kind of exploration should take place.

Again, it is a decision that the parents have to make. As professionals we must be able to guide and support parents and be patient with them during this process. And we must help parents understand that no decision is a final one; that their child's growth must be closely monitored and practices changed to meet the child's changing needs.

My bias, for children who are severely hearing impaired or deaf, is a total communication approach; because I feel that language is developed most effectively with sign.[2] Language input is critical because it is the basis for everything that happens later. The more sophisticated the language and communication skills of the child, the more advanced self awareness, cognition, and social development will be.

I will tell parents what I recommend based on the situation and the hearing loss of the child. If you have a child with a mild, moderate, and sometimes even a severe hearing loss...those kids usually develop good oral language, and you can get them pretty vocal with hearing aids and a good auditory training and language program in the home.

Andy Nielsen:

Assuming the parents have just brought their child in for a hearing test, after informing them of the physical nature of the problem, I would advise them of the long range ramifications.

---

[2]The "total communication" approach mentioned here encourages the use of speech, lip reading, sign language, and finger spelling when communicating with the hard of hearing and the deaf.

It is quite different than the "oral" approach of communication that frowns on the use of sign language and finger spelling, and emphasizes the use of residual hearing and the development of lip reading skills.

The first job would be to surround their child with stimuli for all of his senses. That means getting two good hearing aids on him as soon as possible, and intensifying the total sensory input as much as possible. With a child this young, if the loss is mild or moderate, I would look into an all-in-the-ear type of aid. Later, as the child becomes adapted to the aid, and depending upon the degree of loss, a possible switch to the behind-the-ear type of aid might be appropriate.

In the next four to six weeks I would visit their home and explain the child's problem to as many of the relatives as possible. I would explain how they can all understand the kind of development they will be seeing in the child. If they provide enough extra-sensory input, they are going to see relatively normal development. On the other hand, to start denying and limiting this extra input to the child will limit him developmentally.

The important thing here is to start this extra sensory input immediately. I mean the very day you find out there is a loss, start reinforcing stimuli in a secondary sense. For example, when the child hears a speech sound, make him aware of where it came from. Show him by your facial expressions that you produced the speech sound. Guide the child so that he can feel you make the speech sounds while you are talking to him. If he hears a dog barking, make an effort to allow the child to see the dog barking. If he hears a car horn, let him feel the car and even the horn as it honks.

At six months you are entering into a critical period for language development: the more stimulation you give the child's brain, the more active the brain is going to be, especially in the temporal regions. This will give the child a larger base of information to work with later.

As the parents of a hard of hearing child, you have a child whose information basis is being restricted. If you can use amplification, that will help broaden his information base. If you can give him extra-sensory stimuli, that will do even more to broaden his information base.

Linda Hawbaker:

We had to convince our doctor that there was a problem with Bobby. Our doctor didn't believe it, but we knew it. We knew there was a hearing loss.

We could see Bobby's lack of response to the noises we were making. We saw that he was responding to vibrations or visual stimuli like shadows, but not to auditory stimuli.

When we questioned the doctor, he used the tuning fork method of testing hearing and said Bobby was fine.

But getting back to your original question, I think it is important to introduce the parents to others who are involved in this field. I would let the parents know what kind of services are available to them.

After the physician, a university that has a hearing lab comes to mind. Either the lab or the physician should then be able to give more referrals.

Pauline Zamecki:

Our doctor approached us in a very matter of fact manner. He said, "Your child has a hearing loss." We liked that. It was a straight-forward low key approach, informing us that Paula had a loss.

After that we were given some suggestions on ways that we could get some more information. We were given names of some of the schools in the area that dealt with hearing impairments. Although it was a little early for us to be considering schools for Paula, it was a good referral as we were able to get some support on how to deal with the loss.

The school encouraged us to get hearing aids on Paula as quickly as possible. We were told that six months was not too early. If a baby can hear his own cooing, he will be encouraged to continue cooing, because cooing comes naturally to an infant. Speech development will then be transferred from this cooing relatively easily, compared to the baby who does not have the reinforcement and stops these vocalizations.

As far as the amount of information to give to the parents right away, that depends on the parents. Some parents are ready to go. They want a lot of information as quickly as possible. They want to get on with a program immediately, and actively seek out ideas. Other parents need more time to accept the fact of the hearing loss. Even in the face of the obvious, some will actually deny the fact that there is a loss.

The big thing to remember is that this is not the end of the world! This is just a curve. The child is not lost, he is just hard of hearing. Things are just going to require a little more effort.

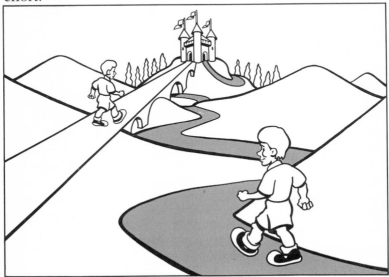

Most of our worries happened before we found out Paula was deaf. We were relieved, as now we knew why things weren't happening; why Paula wasn't answering. There were times that I was really upset, thinking that there might be something really wrong with her mind.

We would have worried a lot more if Paula had been our second child instead of our first. We didn't know it was unusual for her to be sitting and playing in her own little world. We used to brag that she could sleep though anything - just like her Dad! We didn't know that, in fact, she was in her own world. She was not hearing our world. If she had been the second child we would have been a little more suspicious at an earlier stage.

Carolyn Lefever:

I'd want parents to know, that regardless of the age of the onset of the problem, a hard of hearing child will, in all likelihood, become a loner. He or she will not really feel comfortable with either the hearing world or the deaf world for any extended periods of time.

Many hearing people don't want to take the time to do the things needed to help a hard of hearing child to understand. Things like repeating what was said, being sure to face the hard of hearing person, and clarifying the topic of conversation.

Deaf people never really accept hard of hearing people because they hear too much! Sure, a hard of hearing child in a class with deaf children will probably shine in a number of areas such as speech, picking up language and social awareness. But all too often I have seen those children become objects of jealousy, and then be shunned by their deaf classmates.

Even as an adult, I often don't feel that I belong to either group. Deaf people don't accept you because you are not really deaf, and hearing people forget you have trouble and become irritated at having to repeat things.

The parents of a hard of hearing child face some really difficult choices. If they elect to send their child to a regular public school (even with additional help), the day may very well come when she can no longer keep up with regular classes. This usually occurs in late elementary, junior, or senior high school. If the child is then transferred to a deaf school, the child faces the possibility of entering a totally alien world of people communicating with their hands. The frustrations can be enormous. Whatever decisions are made, though, I think the home, and the corresponding language development there, will be the biggest deciding factor in the child's future.

Imagine you have to inform parents that their six-year-old child has been diagnosed hard of hearing. What would you say to them?

Joseph Livingston:

By the time the child is in kindergarten or first grade, you are not going to be informing the parents that their child is deaf or severely hard of hearing, unless their child has just lost his hearing due to a recent infection.

By the time the child is five or six, if the child is severely hard of hearing, and somebody hasn't realized it, something is wrong in the family. We would then have a very different situation than what you would consider a typical family.

You have to deal with the child as an individual. He is a product of the combination of handicaps he has.

I would push a reading and language development program. I think reading and language development are absolutely critical. You just have to push it as far as you can, in every possible way.

Cheryl Deconde Johnson:

Frequently at this stage, the hearing loss is due to an illness such as otitis media, meningitis, or some kind of trauma. Usually a physician is involved as a result of the illness and the child is often hospitalized. However, there are still many children who are hard of hearing and are first diagnosed from initial school screenings.

Most of the kids who have a profound hearing loss are educated in a total communication environment. They can be mainstreamed[3] with the help of an interpreter.

---

[3]The term "mainstreamed" refers to the practice of having hearing impaired children attend classes with normal hearing children. Frequently they are accompanied by an interpreter who will sign the teacher's lecture to the hearing impaired student.

Looking back on my daughter's situation, I wish I had immediately requested a total communication environment even
though she had a significant level of residual hearing. I wish she
had not been limited to auditory-oral input for instruction.
School would have been much less stressful for her.

Communication with children who have acquired a hearing loss later on or have good residual hearing abilities, may
be quite good in the auditory-oral mode because language
structures are generally well established by six years of age.
However, when you are attempting to process more complex information, as you are in an instructional setting, I
don't think its realistic to expect a child to be successful
through the auditory-oral mode alone.

In other words, the communication mode should depend
on the intactness of the auditory system and the quality of
the child's ability to use residual hearing.

More importantly, parents need to be given information
and support to understand and accept their child. They must
be encouraged to communicate with their child in whichev-
er way provides the most meaningful language system. The
importance of developing and preserving the child's self
esteem must be kept in view at all times.

Andrew Nielsen:
You can start by emphasizing to the parents the positive
aspects of a loss that has just been acquired: the child
already has ninety to ninety-five percent of his vocabulary, so
he is going to have a good language base. We are going to
have to work on a maintenance level with speech. For example, there maybe a tendency to loose the pronunciation of
an "s" or something like that with a 50 db loss.

One of the major things we will have to do is help make
the child feel at ease making adjustments for his hearing loss

in school. For example, he is going to have to understand that not all the teachers are going to make sure that he is sitting in the front row of the class. Also the parents will have to understand that they just can't expect a child in the second grade to walk up to the teacher and say, "I am hard of hearing, I need to sit in the front row."

We need to begin preparing the child for puberty by accepting him before adolescence comes on the scene and the differences are accentuated. We must help him make decisions based on what his special needs are going to be.

Don Kitson:

There is a big difference in finding a hearing loss at six years from finding one at six months. I would like to know the child's background. Where was he going to school when he was three years old? Where was he in kindergarten? How did he do?

What to do depends upon the degree of hearing loss. I would suggest leaving the child in the normal classroom programs and watching closely to see if there are any problems. If some problems seem to be developing, then switch the child to an oral-based program. If that doesn't help, then move him to a total communication program that involves mainstreaming.

Imagine you have to inform parents that their twelve-year-old child has been diagnosed hard of hearing. What would you say to them?

Andrew Nielsen:

We are really going to have be on our toes to make sure the child's self-concept emerges intact.

I have more empathy for hard of hearing kids than I do deaf kids. We have to recognize that the hard of hearing child will have the additional problem of trying to decide which world to live in. "At times I am accepted into the hearing world because I can talk, but then at the same time, because I can talk, the deaf world rejects me. One minute the hearing world accepts me, but the next minute the hearing world turns its back on me, because I don't catch a joke. Where do I exist?"

I would hope the parents have already established a good relationship with their child and that they can talk about feelings. When the child comes home from school and he is moody, he is tired, and he feels that the people at school have been laughing at him, is he willing to talk about it?

I think something a hard of hearing child may lose is his sense of humor. So many of our jokes have their real humor in the intonation: what you do with your voice. He is going to have to understand that sometimes people are going to be laughing at a joke, and he is not going to be able to catch it because he was not able to hear the inflection or the intonation. At this point, the child can either fake it by laughing at something he doesn't know anything about, or ask a friend that he is particularly close to for an explanation.

I think another real problem is that sometimes the hard of hearing child who hears the laughter, but not the joke itself, automatically assumes that the laughter is directed at him. It seems that hard of hearing girls are particularly vulnerable to this. I don't know if the boys have some kind of shell or just hold it in, but the girls will frequently just explode in response to situations of this type.

Hard of hearing adolescents will often hear just enough to get themselves into difficult situations. They also have developed enough speech to get themselves into uncomfortable positions. I think a lot of these situations can be avoided. With our middle-school aged kids we spend from 2:30 to 3:20 every Friday, the last hour of class, on what we call debriefing. We talk though the problems the kids have had during the week. For example, we spent four weeks talking about good words that are used in a nasty fashion. There is nothing wrong with the word "suck", used in "I suck my thumb." But in "You suck!", the word has a completely different meaning. If you are in biology class the biology teacher may talk about a "bitch." If you are hard of hearing and your only introduction to this word is "son of a bitch," then there is a real possibility of confusion.

In the afternoon classes there were three profoundly deaf students and five hard of hearing students. For the deaf kids, these classes were almost language development. For the hard of hearing kids, these classes were more likely language clarification.

Linda Storch:

My daughter, Amy, is hard of hearing. I sent her to a regular school and I thought there would be no problem. She had no special teacher's aide with her.

When she was eleven years old she became confused. She wanted to play sports, but she felt left out. She felt bad if the hearing children said to her, "Never mind" or "Forget it," in response to her questions. She felt hurt. She felt the other girls did not accept her, so she had a hard time accepting herself.

Last year she really had a hard time. She was very frustrated. She would ask me what the teachers said about her. She became afraid of the teachers and of the hearing children.

This fall I placed Amy in a deaf school and she is much happier. The problem now is that her academic level is above her peers, and I don't feel she is getting the necessary challenge. She is getting A's and B's.

I am not completely happy with the situation. On one hand, my hard of hearing daughter is happier socially and emotionally in a deaf school because she can communicate with her peers, but academically she is not getting challenged. Though she is in eighth grade, most of her deaf friends are in high school.

I would like her to return to a regular classroom, but she is adamant in her refusal.

Pauline Zamecki:

The parents have to know that how they accept the new situation will have a very strong influence on how the child will accept the situation. This is more true now than when the child was six years old.

The child is going to take a reading of mom and dad right away. If they seem to be scared or ashamed of his problem, then the child will be scared or ashamed also. The parents are going to have to get their act together immediately - that twelve year old needs their support.

The child will be better off now than if the loss had occurred at six months of age. At least now the speech and language development are intact. So to a great extent the hard of hearing child will be limited only by the degree the parents think he is going to be limited.

Imagine you have to inform parents that their six-month-old, six-year-old, or twelve-year-old child has been diagnosed as being deaf, not hard of hearing. What would you say to them?

Joe Livingston:

To a degree, the response will be the same here as with the first question in that I want the family to seek professional help. Whenever you are informing people about something that is attacking their children, you better do it very, very carefully... with an awful lot of empathy. They need your support, they need guidance, they need help. If you don't do it in a way that shows them your level of genuine concern for them, you will lose them. They will go someplace else and critical time will be wasted.

You have to get them working on the problem, rather than just worrying about diagnosing the problem. By accepting the problem, I do not mean not looking for a correct diagnosis. But after the diagnosis has been reasonably established the parents need to move on to finding solutions.

The biggest thing is understanding the implications of a diagnosis of deafness. If we are talking about a first born six-month-old child from a family that has never had contact with the deaf world before, we are talking about a large adjustment. The parents have no concept of what is ahead.

For example, they have no concept of how language is acquired. They don't understand what it means not to hear. This whole process requires a tremendous amount of learning on the parents' part.

Andy Nielsen:

A lot of people see hearing losses as being gradient. I see hearing losses as either pre-language or post-language. I would say the approach would be totally different, although it may seem that I am saying the same thing but for different reasons. Comparing a hard of hearing child and a deaf child is like comparing apples and oranges, they are just not the same.

With a deaf child, I would prepare the parents for the idea that they have a unique child. There is potential for your child and if you follow these steps, then your child is going to enjoy a fairly normal development as long as you don't try to make him a pale imitation of a hearing person. Respect his dignity as a deaf individual.

Understand that he is probably going to gravitate towards a different culture than yours as he grows older...and that is going to be good for you and good for him. But encourage him to understand that for every aspect of his life, other than his social and emotional life, he will be working with hearing people, and he had better learn to understand hearing people.

Even at six months of age we have to start working toward this goal. We are going to have him play football with hearing kids, and we are going to be taking him down to the arts fair to compete with hearing kids. We are going to show him that he can compete on almost every level with hearing people.

Obviously some areas will be closed. If he is four years old and says he wants to fly an airplane that is fine. But if he is profoundly deaf and thinks he is going to be a commercial airline pilot, we are in trouble.[4]

You don't take a hard of hearing or deaf child and deny him the right to fail. He has the right to try and the right to fail. A large percentage of life is adjusting to failure.

---

[4]Author's note: There are approximately fifty certified deaf pilots in the United States, although they do not fly in a commercial capacity. The author, who is deaf in his right ear and hard of hearing in his left ear, is a former Flight Instructor and an active pilot.

Going back to the six-month-old deaf child, we are going to do a lot of the same things as with the hard of hearing child: we are going to use amplification; we are going to get the parents involved in a sign language class as fast as possible, preferably in a morpheme-based[5] type of sign language. Then when the child gets to be four, five or six years of age, we are going to start going to adult deaf activities once or twice a month. We are hearing parents, but we are going to take our deaf child into his world once or twice a month. As he grows and has developed his morpheme-based sign language, we are going to teach him American Sign Language (ASL),[6] which he is going to learn to use in these settings.

Now, as much as I respect the deaf culture and as much as I respect the American Sign Language as a system of communication, until an English language based signing system is used, at least in our classrooms, I do not think we will see an appreciable increase in the academic performance of our deaf students. Understand that I am talking about an across-the-board perspective. We can always point to the 2 to 5 percent of the deaf community that go to Gallaudet (a college for the deaf that uses ASL American Sign Language) and say,

---

[5] A "morpheme-based" type of sign language usually involves a system of signs in which even the smallest meaningful language unit has a sign movement assigned to it. For example, the word "misunderstanding" would conceivably involve four sign movements: one each for "mis", "under", "stand", and "ing."

[6] American Sign Language (ASL) is a means of communication that is based upon the use of finger spelling, signs, and gestures to convey the meaning of an idea. The emphasis is on concepts and does not necessarily follow the rules of syntax of the English language. One gesture can contain the same information as an entire English sentence.

An encoded English-based system of sign language is a more recent development of signs that is based upon the use of finger spelling, signs, and a sentence structure that more closely follows the patterns of the English language. Although both methods will sometimes use the same signs, they are quite different sign language systems.

"Look at the great job they are doing." But let's look at the sixty to seventy percent of the deaf adults that are employed well below their ability level...I think the major reason for this is their lack of English language development.

I can not confirm this, but I remember hearing of a situation where one of the big things in a certain state was teaching the kids at the high school level how to apply for SSI.[7] I think this is very wrong. I think this is a way to teach a person to be crippled, to say it is okay to take your four hundred bucks a month, tax free, add food stamps, and without working, clear approximately seven hundred dollars a month! To my knowledge this can go on indefinitely. To me that is an absolute insult to humanity.

Now, I can see SSI programs as beneficial if you use that money to enrich the child's life. If I was part of a middle income family and I could get an extra one hundred twenty dollars a month for my child to provide him with some extra experiences... For example, deaf students can not go into the armed forces, so they can not receive veteran's benefits to further a college education. So I am comfortable with deaf students applying their SSI to college tuition.

Helga Simpson:
In my case, there was never anybody in my family who was deaf or had become deaf. It was quite a shock to me. I would try to tell the parents to accept the situation as quickly as possible. Try not to convey to the child your own fears of what is ahead. Get in touch with the closest school for advice.

I got in touch with the John Tracy Clinic when Jenny was six months old and they were a great help. Because Jenny

[7]Supplemental Security Income available from the federal government to the handicapped. It can continue for life.

was profoundly deaf, I quickly came to the conclusion that I would have to learn sign language to communicate with my daughter. I strongly recommend the use of sign language for any child who is profoundly deaf, so the child can communicate with the parents and the world.

Treat the child just like any other child. Try to be there for that child, but no more than for any other child unless, of course, there is some emergency.

The child that becomes deaf at a later age, say six years, has the big advantage of already having the basics of language.

If the deafness occurs even later, say twelve years of age, there is going to be some need of counseling. The child at the age of twelve is very aware of peer pressure, and it would be difficult for a child this age to accept deafness.

The child would probably resist wearing a new hearing aid and might even hide it. It would probably be more difficult for the twelve-year-old child to adjust to this situation than for the six year old.

Pauline Zamecki:

The parents of a deaf child would greatly benefit from experiencing silence for a while. Try a set of headphones that deafen sound. Try watching TV without any volume. Many times, as parents, we feel the child is not listening because they don't want to; but a deaf child may be ignoring you because he can't hear what you are saying.

Richard Zamecki:

I would stress that the children learn to lip-read and to use their voices. Sign alone is not enough. They need the lip-reading experiences and the voice experiences. We did not

learn sign language and Paula had to watch our lips. If that
didn't work then we had to write it out on paper. Paula
didn't learn sign language until she was eleven years old.

Pauline Zamecki:

If the child was older and the deafness resulted from an
accident or sudden illness, I would advise some counseling
for both the parents and the child. This situation could scare
the child to death.

We know of a girl that Paula went to school with who
thought her hearing would improve as she became older
because her sisters were older and they could hear.

Some older children who have lost their hearing will wonder if this is some kind of punishment for something they
have done. There will be a lot of emotional trauma at this
age. Not only is there a loss of hearing but there is a loss of
communication. This is scary and frustrating. You feel very
much alone.

Sheila Kidder:

As with the hard of hearing child, put the hearing aids on
as quickly as possible. In addition, you have to teach them to
learn to listen. Even if the child is deaf, every little sound he
can get helps.

If the child has not heard, then he doesn't know how to
listen and connect the sound with a meaning. He must learn
to connect listening to meaning. Deaf children need it all:
the hearing aids, the sign language, the association with
other children who are deaf, and the association with other
children who have normal hearing.

In regular public schools the deaf are different. Many times
this creates emotional problems. In their own schools they

are with a group of children who have the same difficulty. They can excel within their own group. Here they can build their self-confidence. Then they can go out and compete with others. True, formal education is important, but if the deaf do not have a good social atmosphere they are not going to excel anywhere. Get them into a school where they can associate and compete with other children like themselves.

Carolyn Lefever:

With a deaf child, language and communication are the key to the future. With the very young child, I would do everything I could to make the parents see that they must begin communicating immediately. My preference for this is total communication - signing in English, and emphasizing speech and speech reading as they get older. Deafness requires a total change in the life of the family. It is, sadly, a dedication and effort that a lot of families seem unwilling or unable to make.

A child who becomes deaf later in some ways faces a greater ordeal: most families do not adjust themselves to the loss and the youngster often withdraws into a shell.

What symptoms would you look for if you suspected that a child was hard of hearing or deaf?

Linda Hawbaker:

When Bobby was a baby, we would enter his room and open and shut the door. Bobby would not react to the noise. He would still be looking in the same direction as when we walked in. When we were in the kitchen, we could rattle pots and pans like crazy and Bobby would not respond.

The doctor who delivered Bobby, had recently delivered another boy who had lost his hearing due to meningitis. When we kept mentioning to him that we felt something was wrong with Bobby's hearing, he had a hard time accepting the idea. These would have been the only two kids this age, who were deaf, in a whole town of 40,000 people. I think the doctor had a hard time dealing with this emotionally.

It took some of our friends, who happened to be teachers of the deaf, to recommend that we take Bobby to get a professional evaluation of his hearing. We took him to an audiology clinic at a university for repeated tests. We found that he had a profound hearing loss due to nerve deafness.

Later we started to notice other things. Bobby didn't walk until he was sixteen months old. We also noticed that he had very difficult time seeing at dusk. We asked people about this, but nobody made any connection between the two or with the hearing problem.

It was only after I saw a movie about retinitis pigmentosa,[8] which described the type of vision loss peculiar to

---

[8]This is a degenerative condition of the retina of unknown cause. It is a progressive impairment of visual function that usually manifests itself in childhood. The first sympton is an impairment of night vision. Daytime vision can deteriorate to the point where there is a profound loss.

that disease, that I suddenly was aware of what Bobby had. Bobby does have some constriction of the blood vessels in his eyes. Our doctor says they have not deteriorated since he started seeing Bobby six years ago, so there seems to be no further deterioration at this point. There is always the possibility that this could start to change and he could develop tunnel vision or even become blind.

We believe his problems are due to Usher's Syndrome.[9] It is very difficult to pinpoint because there are many different types of Usher's Syndrome. Now there is a screening for this kind of a loss. The prognosis remains an individual thing.

Pam Pflueger:

Does the child respond to one parent's voice more often than the other? It is possible that he finds it easier to hear one frequency range better than the other. Does the child seem to be watching your lips rather than hearing your voice? Cover your mouth with your hand or a napkin and see how your child responds when you address him. Does your child seem to nod his head, and yet not respond in an appropriate manner when asked a question or given a direction? Does your child seem to respond only to those sounds that project vibrations? Does his speech and language development seem to be delayed? Does his voice have an unusual tone? Is it nasal or high pitched? Does your child demonstrate poor balance or poor motor coordination? Does the child have a short attention span or isolate himself from other children?

---

[9]Usher's syndrome is a condition that has the symptoms of retinitis pigmentosa and the additional complications of a profound loss of hearing.

Patty Pittroff Swain:

The first thing my mother noticed with me was that I was not talking. Until the age of three I seemed to be responding and talking in a normal manner. Then things changed. I stopped talking. I did not respond when my back was turned to my mother. I was also not really playing with other children. I had quietly withdrawn into my own world.

Pauline Zamecki:

One thing I would look for is hyperactivity in the child: the child might be trying to catch everything with his eyes.

Also, don't be afraid to check things out. Sometimes when you are with a child from day to day you don't notice things that an impartial observer might notice right away. If a friend of yours suggests that your child might be having a hearing problem at least check it out. Don't become defensive about it. It is nothing to be defensive about. Just check out the possibility.

I remember a friend of mine who kept complaining that she couldn't control her son. I asked her if son's hearing had been checked. She responded yes, and the doctors said there was nothing wrong. Well, I was so worried in light of my own experiences with Paula, that I later called her and gave her some phone numbers of some people who could recheck her son's hearing.

About a year later I met this mother at Paula's school, and she came up to me and thanked me. As it turned out her son did have a hearing loss, and after putting hearing aids on the child, he had become an entirely different boy. Bad professional advice can cause a lot of problems.

Sheila Kidder:

For the hard of hearing child I would notice the speech. Usually the child, depending upon the severity of the loss, will have some speech impairment. Also the attention span may be very short.

Shannon, our deaf daughter, did not make any of the cooing sounds that our other children made. The only sounds Shannon made were laughter and crying.

When my other children were very young I was able to calm them down by cradling and talking to them. But Shannon never seemed to calm down when I talked to her. She would accept being held, but my cooing never seemed to have that calming effect.

I remember taking Shannon to a pediatrician when she was six months old. He tested her hearing by clicking his fingers near one side of her head and then doing the same thing on the other side. She responded to the movement of his hand - not to the noise of his fingers. The doctor told us there was nothing wrong with her, take her home and leave her alone. Shannon was a bright child. She was able to compensate very well for her deafness. But, still, we felt that something was not right.

Then when Shannon was about twelve months old, I remember a friend of ours visited us with her baby boy. He was two weeks older than Shannon. They were playing together. They were doing all the same things. But when one of us would make a noise, my friend's boy would turn around and Shannon would not. So we got a big metal pan and spoon and started banging the two together behind the children. Shannon would not respond. This is when we knew darn well that somebody was crazy and it wasn't us!

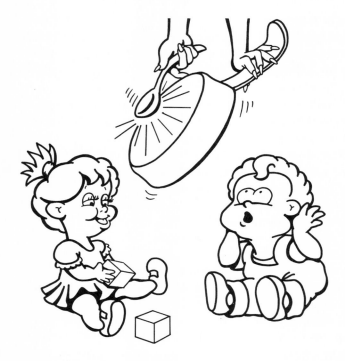

Finally, at thirteen months of age we took her to an oto-laryngologist. We found the problem. We immediately put a hearing aid on her and started her in an auditory training program with the John Tracy Clinic.

If one is to raise a deaf or hard of hearing child in an oral program, what criteria does one use to judge it successful? At what stage in the child's development does one decide to change to a total program, if at all?[10]

Joseph Livingston:

You stay on top of it from day one, and you plan some landmarks you are going to look for. For instance, what kind of language should my child have by one, two, and three years of age? Measurement could be expressed in terms of the number of words in the expressive vocabulary, the reading level, the language structure, and all the other areas that pertain to language development.

If you find the child is not learning what he should, then you need to look into the possibilities of changing the program. You really can't wait until the child is twelve years old to make this change.

Hopefully you will have a professional working with you who knows the stages of language growth and can guide you as to whether they are being achieved. If the professional doesn't know anything about these stages, then I strongly suggest you seek the advise of another professional who does. When a professional sees that growth is not being made, then I would hope he would then reevaluate the program.

If the communication mode needs to be changed, so be it. I really don't give a hoot which mode is used as long as the communication is getting through to the child. The communication system doesn't make any difference in itself, it is

---

[10]At the risk of being redundant, an "oral program" focuses on the use of the residual hearing of the individual. Emphasis is placed on the development of lip reading and speech skills. Sign language would not be a part of such a program.

A "total program" would encompass all the parts of an oral program, with the addition of sign language and finger spelling.

what you are doing with it that makes the difference. Is it working successfully in the development of language?

Success is a relative thing. By three years of age, you should have words strung together in sequences. You should have good multi-level linguistic expressive language. The speech quality itself is not so important to me, as seeing the use of good vocabulary and sentence structures.

By five years of age you should see dramatic increases in the child's language and the start of a good reading program. By seven years of age there should a measurable reading program. If these things are not present, find another program.

Again, if you don't see very strong growth in language by three years of age I would question the program. You can not hesitate to insure that your child has a good and successful language development program. Time is not on your side.

Cheryl Deconde Johnson:

Personally, I feel that a total communication program offers so much more, right from the start, that I would usually recommend it. I understand that for various reasons some parents and families will want to put their child in an oral program.

I am reminded of a family that had started their child, who had a severe/profound hearing loss, in an oral program in a regular school. She was in fourth grade and she was really struggling. The parents knew it, the teachers knew it, and she knew it. She just wasn't getting enough of the content. The FM phonic ear amplification system wasn't enough.[11] The information in the classroom was so complex and was given out so quickly that she was not able to absorb it.

---

[11]The FM amplification system is a system where the teacher (or a parent) will use a microphone that transmits an FM signal to a receiver that is a part of a body-style hearing aid. This type of aid can be set to receive and amplify only FM transmissions of the microphone, thereby eliminating any extraneous environmental noises that might interfere with the message.

She was doing okay in the mainstreamed classroom socially, but she needed an interpreter who could sign the instruction to fill in the information she missed. Once this was provided (after some sign language instruction) she was able to comprehend and perform much better. Each child needs to be looked at individually. Would this child benefit from a manual sign language system? If so, why not use it? If there is no need, then that is fine, too.

The key is the family, the parents. Are they willing to look at the situation realistically and are they willing to commit themselves to a total communication program, if it is deemed to be in the best interest of the child and his education? To work, the total communication program has to be accepted and supported by the parents. Many times this decision is not made in five minutes. It takes some exploration and it takes some time.

Parents should not feel locked into anything. Services should be under constant review. When a particular method or strategy is not working, modifications must be made. Realistic goals and expectations are extremely important to developing successful programs for children.

You don't always know what a child will be able to do when he is two years of age. The child may progress well with an oral approach, and then again he may require a system that includes the use of signs.

My personal feeling is that if you start out using signs, you increase the amount of language the child is receiving. Time is very critical in the early years. When input is restricted, language acquisition will be greatly hampered, resulting in significant language delay which is rarely overcome.

I see no detriment to the use of sign language. I get asked about that frequently, even with kids who are hard of hearing rather than deaf. Will signing harm them by limiting the development of their auditory skills and speech production? No.

In our preschool we have kids who are hard of hearing. They are usually quite vocal when they enter the program. Often we see their vocalizations decrease dramatically during the first few weeks they are in the program. This occurs because the children are taking in a new method of communication, the use of signs. We have to prepare parents for this. It doesn't mean the child has lost his speech, it is just that his focus has temporarily changed. The verbal expressions come back after this initial focusing is diffused into other learning.

Andrew Nielsen:

I personally feel a completely oral approach is in reality a denial of the problem. As long as the parents and teachers of this approach don't deny the deafness, and they realize that at some point in time they very well might have to go to a visual language system, then fine, give it a try.

Personally, my answer to your question, "When would I change to a total communication program?", is as soon as the hearing loss has been identified.

Don Kitson:

Many times, when the parents have their child in an oral program, they expect the child to be normal. Most oral programs start at the preschool level and continue until eighth grade. I have never seen an oral program start at the ninth grade level.

I would wait until the child is six or eight years of age to make any changes from an oral program. I was raised in an oral situation myself and didn't learn sign language until I was in college.

Yita Harrison:

Is the child learning in the oral program? Is he improving? Is he functioning up to the level that should be expected of him? Is he motivated in his learning? If not, I personally would not waste time. As soon as you suspect the answers to these questions are not satisfactory, move immediately into a total communication program.

You have to remember that, from the very beginning, the hearing impaired child is from three to five years behind his hearing peers in getting vocabulary and language input. If you do not see any progress with an oral program then change immediately. You do not have the luxury of wasting any more time.

Linda Hawbaker:

I would want to see progress in language development and reading skills. If the child enters the third grade and is not reading at the first grade level it is time for a change. You can't wait until the fifth grade, as the gulf in the reading levels will be too large. I would make a change in educational placement no later than the third grade.

Larry Hawbaker:

I don't see the profoundly deaf ever being fully served in an oral program. If there is a profound deafness I would go to the total communication program immediately.

If there is a more moderate loss then I would perhaps start out in an oral program, but monitor the progress or lack thereof very closely. If it is not working, don't hesitate to change.

Tutoring can make a difference in speech. We had a speech tutor for Bobby for a while, but this is a luxury most people can not afford. Also, there is a question as to how much of that speech is retained in understandable speech after the training ceases.

Linda Hawbaker:

Speech is a learned skill. It is difficult to retain without years of intense one-on-one training and reinforcement. Frequently it stops, or diminishes greatly, after the training stops.

Larry Hawbaker:

With a hard of hearing person the speech training would probably be a lot more beneficial. Depending upon the degree of loss, I would also support the use of sign language to cover any educational gaps that might occur if one were to rely on speech alone.

Helga Simpson:

I would compare the progress of the child to the progress of children in regular schools for any particular grade level. If the progress is not there, get into a total program - fast.

As to when, it depends upon the child. Is the child happy in the present environment? Does the child show any fear of asking questions in an oral environment? If the child is not happy, change immediately.

Pam Pflueger:

I would ask the parents to explore their answers to the some of the following questions:

1. Is your child increasing his vocabulary?

2. Is he increasing his reading and language levels? Does he seem to enjoy reading?

3. Is his speech improving?

4. Is he able to define the words that he can say and use them appropriately?

5. Academically how far behind is your child from other hearing children his age?

6. In class how far behind other deaf children is your child?

7. How well can your child understand written and oral directions from you and from people who are not members of his immediate family?

8. How comfortable do you feel exploring and explaining a concept with your child?

9. How well can your child talk to you and explain his feelings and thoughts?

10. If a total program is being considered, in addition to the auditory/speech training, are you willing to learn sign language?

If you don't feel you can answer most of the previous questions in a positive manner and your child has been in an oral setting for a year or two, I would consider switching to a total communication setting. Be aware that time is especially critical for a child who has not developed a language base due to a congenital hearing loss. Even if a language base has been established, I would continue to emphasize auditory and speech training.

Richard Zamecki:

Get involved in finding children who are in this program and see how they are doing. Do they measure up to what you feel your child should be doing when your child reaches that age?

I would contact the parents and talk with them. The school, of course, is going to show you their best students. Meet with a variety of parents to get a more realistic picture of where their children are going with the program.

Not everybody can get involved. But just because others can't get involved in evaluating a program, doesn't mean you can't become involved. How good do you want this program to be for your child? Most of the time you really have to organize and fight for quality. It will not be just handed to you.

Pauline Zamecki:

That is true with any program. If you want your child to be better, then you are going to have to work with that in mind. You have to decide whether you want to work eighteen years of your life, to make your child's next fifty years better.

Richard Zamecki:

Getting back to your original question, Paula changed into a total communication program when she was eleven. I am glad she had the oral background, but do believe this all depends upon the individual child.

Pauline Zamecki:

This is true. If you see a child stagnating in his educational growth, regardless of age, I would recommend changing communication approaches.

Some of the other students in Paula's oral program never developed any speech skills. They never said, "Mom." They never said, "ball." Not one word. They waited until the kids were in junior high before they were introduced to a signed communication system. That is ridiculous. These kids should have been learning sign language in a total communication program as soon as it became apparent that they were not going to succeed in an oral environment. Professionals should know this.

Richard Zamecki:

Paula was able to learn in an oral program. She was bright enough to do it. I recognize that not all kids will be able to do that. I supported Paula being in a oral program because I wanted her to develop her speech skills to the maximum. Also, I didn't want to learn sign language. Maybe I was just being lazy and selfish, but I don't regret the oral emphasis given to Paula. I think she functions in the hearing world a lot better because of it.

I think if you learn sign first, then it is the easy way out. You will not have to develop any speech reading skills, or speech itself, because the signs will help you communicate more easily. Everybody will take the easy way out. Since trying to communicate with signs is easier than using speech skills, there is no incentive for kids to learn speech skills if they have acquired the use of sign language.

Pauline Zamecki:

I disagree. Sign language is not necessarily the easy way out. Sign language is not universal. Signing requires a lot of effort.

Communication is the bottom line. Whatever is necessary to communicate successfully should be used. If it requires standing on your head, then so be it.

Richard Zamecki:

Well, that is fine, but I still believe that to develop the use of speech skills, sign language should be held off for several years. This was done with Paula and I think this is why Paula has developed the speech skills she has. ·

I agree, with signs you could have communicated with her easier. But the speech development would not have been there.

Pauline Zamecki:

If she would have been exposed to a universal sign language at an earlier age, and the signs would have been in exact English, I believe her reading skills would have been a lot better. She would have been able to see what she read. It would have been a part of her normal life.

Unfortunately, there are a lot of different variations in sign language. It is not universal. Most are not set forth in exact English. It is difficult to transfer this non-English syntax to written English.

Sheila Kidder:

Evaluate the vocabulary. Evaluate the speech. Evaluate the sentence structure.

Most of the deaf that do well in oral programs fall into one of two categories. Either they are only moderately hearing impaired, or they have not had a life of their own. The latter group grew up on the speech chair. Frequently, the successful ones are found in one-child families where the parents have the time and resources to devote everything to this one child.

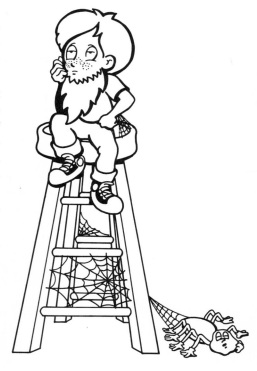

I do not feel that the profoundly deaf do that well in an oral program. There are too many sounds that look alike. Words can be interchanged so easily and this can be very confusing.

I would say within a one year period you should have seen definite progress in a particular program. Perhaps the answer may not be to abandon the program, but to add to it. Add the use of signs. The best is to give them both a speech program and a sign program.

Shannon was in an oral program until she was four. At that point we were just about ready to send her to a residential school. She didn't understand what I wanted. I didn't understand what she wanted. We both were going out of our minds. It was a wrestling match every time we wanted to get her to do anything.

The oral school had us practice for six months on the word "ball." They thought that was fine progress.

To give you an example of the way this school handled things, when it was time for the children's ear molds to be made, the teachers could not explain to the children what was happening. So they prepared for the worst by having a teacher hold each child's legs and arms while the molds were being made. Needless to say, the next time the children saw an ear mold session being readied, they thought it was time for a fight. This lack of communication and use of force made Shannon fearful of and angry at anything involving medicine.

One time she struck a car - she actually ran out to hit a car. When we took her to the hospital, the doctor wanted to take her temperature. We literally had to strap her down so he could do that. It was all because we could not communicate with her.

Ron Kidder:

If you have seen the movie about Helen Keller, titled *The Miracle Worker,* that was just the way it was. There were a lot of fights until we switched from an oral program to a total communication program that used sign language. Once the communication paths were open, the difference was like night and day.

Sheila Kidder:

The problem we were having in the oral program was that during the parent meeting we were all told that we would be crazy to allow our child to learn sign language. We were told the oral approach was the only way to go; there was no other way. We didn't know of any alternative. Besides who were we to judge? We were not the professionals in the field of deaf education. They had us so brain-washed that we couldn't see what was happening. Just because you are talking with professionals, doesn't mean they are always right. Very rarely does a professional know the child better than a parent knows the child.

But a lot of people are intimidated by professionals. I know we were. For several years we went through an awful time listening to this advice. If things do not seem to be going right, don't hesitate to question the wisdom of a program.

A parent comes to you and asks whether her child should learn sign language. How would you respond?

Joseph Livingston:

I would not feel comfortable answering this question until I had some more background information about the child. I would need to know the child and how the child was functioning. I would need to know the degree of hearing loss. I would want to know the age of the child. How has speech development progressed with the child? I would want to know why the parent is asking me this question. Where is the parent coming from?

If you mean that sign language is to be the primary means of communication, well that is a whole different ball game than simply having the knowledge of signs and using sign language as a secondary means of communication. Both of my daughters sign and both of my daughters are hearing.

If, for example, the child is six years of age and has not developed a viable means of communication through speech, then you better start another means of communication and do it quickly.

I do think it is important that you don't give blanket advice. Advice needs to be tailored to a specific individual and a specific family's ability to get involved with different programs. It does no good to learn sign language if there is nobody to sign to. The sign language communication between the parent and the child would be a start, but in order to develop language the child must be able to communicate with more people. I feel that if the situation is one in which the family is in a small community where nobody uses sign language, then the language will not develop.

I think it is important for the parents to move to a community that has a good educational program for their child. Then they can see their options more clearly. Then the parents can make a decision as to whether sign language is appropriate.

Cheryl Deconde Johnson:
The oral approach has some limitations. I think this is because speech is so hard for some children to learn. Due to the severity of the hearing loss, the sounds required for speech are not clear. When they are learning to talk, there are no references for them for the sounds they should be producing.

From my own experience as a parent, my biggest frustration with my daughter was communication. If we had used sign language, it would have alleviated a lot of the behavior problems and stress that occurred when we were trying to rely on verbal communication alone.

My daughter did not start in a hearing impaired program until she was in kindergarten. I had tried to get her enrolled in a preschool total communication program, but the staff felt she did not have enough of a hearing impairment to warrant being in a total communication environment.

Looking back, I feel you can combine sign language and oral communication into an effective program at a young age. It would eliminate so much of the frustration both parents and child have when they can't get their ideas across to each other. With the use of sign language, ideas can be exchanged very, very quickly. And this is the key in life - communication.

In our program we try to encourage the parents to learn sign language as quickly as possible. We have a home program that starts with the children from identification to three years of age. When the child is ready, at about two and a half years, we bring her into our day preschool program.

Certainly if the child has severe or profound hearing impairment, I strongly support the use of sign language. I also support the use of a manually encoded English type of system as opposed to an American Sign Language type of system.

I know there is a lot of controversy in the deaf community about these two systems. I personally feel that until deaf children learn English, their literacy, whether it is oral or written, is going to be poor.

"You say what you hear." In the deaf world you say what you see. If you constantly see only thoughts and concepts in your visual communication, that is how you are going to write, think, and speak. I do think American Sign Language is a valid language of its own, and there is place for it as such.

On the other hand, if the deaf child is constantly seeing the English language as hearing people use it, but in a visual system that is manually encoded, then he will more likely write, think, and communicate in idiomatic English. For children in an educational setting this is most appropriate.

Frequently, we teach American Sign Language to hearing impaired students in high school as a secondary language. Our students can then communicate with the older members of the deaf community. It will be interesting to see what happens in the future as more children leave school with fully developed English language sign skills.

I do think that not only the parents but grandparents and other members of the family benefit from learning sign language. I have seen parents make video tapes of signs and then mail them to their parents and relatives. The use of video should provide many new opportunities for teaching and developing sign language skills at all levels.

Andrew Nielsen:

If the child is hard of hearing, he could gain a lot from the use of on interpreter in a crowd. Of course, in the classroom this is a great benefit. Sign language with a deaf child is language development.

I have never seen a study that indicated that a child learning to sign loses some of his ability to speak. I have seen situations where the child is expected to be verbal, and this has diminished his language development. It depends upon the amount of hearing loss. For up to a 40 to 50 db loss it is hard to give a general answer. A lot will depend upon the individual child and his environment.

I learned sign language because I saw that my son, Joel, was not making it. At the time Joel was six years of age. We started finger-spelling and later went into signs. At the time Joel was in an oral program, but there were too many frustrations for him and for us.

Pam Pflueger:

The answer to this question depends upon the individual child. If sign is used, a total approach is necessary which includes speech and auditory training. Sign language can give you the means to explain vocabulary and concepts with less of a struggle. If sign language is used, I do feel that Signing Exact English is preferable to American Sign Language for instructional purposes. It is easier to train students to learn how to speak and attend to different sounds while using Signing Exact English. In my classroom I always used my voice while signing and expected the same from my students.

I know some students who learned sign language and then felt they didn't need to use speech. They preferred to associate with their deaf friends who chose not to speak and I understand that.

But one must consider ways of communicating with hearing people also. My brother's good speech and speech reading skills[12] have enabled him to get along well in the work environment. His co-workers who hear him feel comfortable when talking with him.

My parents were told that if they permitted my brother to learn sign language he would never speak. That is a frightening absolute to give parents.

My brother was then enrolled in an intensive auditory, speech, and speech reading training program. While he did excel in these particular areas, his reading vocabulary seemed to be limited. There were also times when it was difficult for him to identify words to express his feelings.

When he was sixteen he was permitted to learn sign language and it became easier for him to expand and improve his reading vocabulary. At first he didn't like it: here he was, sixteen and doing something different. He didn't want to be different than hearing teenagers. Later, he saw how much easier it was for him to communicate with sign language and he accepted it. I should add that he is more comfortable using sign language when he is among a group of people who also sign.

He continued to rely on his speech reading and auditory skills, and would compliment these skills with the sign language he was learning. He did not lose his speech habits because our family was very adamant that he continue to develop his speech. I feel that his learning sign language did not hamper his speech, but served to bolster language development.

Communication between the child and the parents is a two-way street. For communication using sign language to be successful, parents need to take an active role in learning sign language, too.

---

[12]The terms "speech reading" and "lip reading" are used interchangeably.

If your child is in an educational setting where signing is permitted, do evaluate the subject matter being taught. My brother's first experience with total communication was less than satisfactory: the students were treated as if they were in a class of failures. It was taught as a basic learning skills class, which proved to be very limiting. Demand excellence not only in the method of communication, but in what is being taught.

Patty Pittroff Swain:

Depending upon the progress of the child in school, I would introduce sign language. I was very frustrated in school. I missed out on a lot. I did not learn sign language until I was in college. I was a lot happier then, but there were many times I still felt lost.

I was not completely deaf but I could not hear well either. I was not a part of either world. Many hard of hearing children feel as I did.

I am a firm believer in the total communication approach: give the children as much communication as possible. I have never seen a situation where the learning of sign language hampered the development of speech. I think that is just some silly philosophy from a strict one-method group of educators.

Paula Smith:

The longer I work in the field of deaf education, the more I am convinced that children with severe or profound hearing losses need sign language. They miss so many of the auditory clues, that they do not get enough language input. Even with a language training program at home, many of the children are just not capable of absorbing the stimuli without using sign language.

I believe in a total communication program. The child who has the capabilities to develop speech should be encouraged to do so, reinforced by the language development that sign language offers. Even if the hard of hearing child demonstrated good progress in speech and language development up to the age of three, I would still consider the use of sign language as a back-up system for later academic programs.

Yita Harrison:

That's a tough one. I firmly believe in total communication. Over the years that I have been teaching, I have seen many children from oral backgrounds. The parents are happy when they hear their child say, "Mother," but do the children really understand what they are saying?

There is a tremendous difference between children who started with a total communication program, and those who started with an oral program and only later were introduced to total communication. Those who started in a total communication program were way ahead in language development.

I have also seen situations where some of our students would leave our total communication environment and try a mainstream approach. They would come back having retained little or nothing from their mainstreaming. I question whether they really received any meaningful input at all.

I believe the most important thing is that the kids get help at home. This means communication, and really, communication is a two way street. I have had some parents come up to me and ask, "What is wrong with my child? He is always complaining." Frequently, I find that the child is sick, and I have to interpret between the child and the parents. Why can't the parents make the effort to learn sign language? They could then have easily understood the problem themselves and taken their child to a doctor. I think it is terribly unfortunate that many parents can not communicate with their own children.

Linda Hawbaker:

Before Bobby learned sign language life was hell. Bobby would run and point towards a cabinet while he was crying and we had no idea what he was trying to tell us. His behavior was horrendous. After we started using signs, life changed tremendously. So we would automatically say, "Yes, learn sign language right away." Bobby started learning sign language just before he was two. We both learned sign language, because we felt it would make a difference in Bobby's language and reading development. We believe it has. Signing Exact English[13] allows us to do language modeling with Bobby. He can not hear the English language, but he can see it.

Signing Exact English is a lot of work. It is much harder than using signs in a general way to get a concept across. The closer we get to signing idiomatic English, the easier it is for the child to see the English language. I believe this can only help when it comes to language and reading development.

At the same time we want to emphasize that the word "total" in a "total communication approach" also means speech development. Both oral and manual communication avenues need to be encouraged. Though there is no negative to learning sign language, there is the danger of not emphasizing speech development at the same time.

---

[13]"Signing Exact English" is the name of a sign language system being used extensively in the western United States. It has several variations, some demanding the signing of the smallest morpheme components of individual words. In one form or another it requires the signing of each word in the English language as it would normally be spoken or written.

Actually we feel that the signing of idiomatic English encourages the development of speech. The language and words that are visually present then encourage a transfer to the speech mode.

We have an interesting story about that. Bobby has a hearing nephew who is about a year old. Even though his nephew can not speak yet, he has learned some basic signs. He is able to communicate his needs to Bobby even though he can't talk. It shows us again that the use of sign language can eliminate a lot of the frustrations when either speech or hearing is not functioning.

Pauline Zamecki:

Communication is the name of the game. I don't care how is it done. Paula went through a lot of emotional trauma that she would not have had to go through if we could have communicated more easily.

Richard Zamecki:

I have observed that when a child uses sign language with others who also use sign language (often people in the non-hearing world), the child stops using his voice. Even worse, when he is young, he does not develop the use of his voice. Then he is stuck in the deaf culture because he hasn't developed any other mode of communication, except the use of signs. He can't go out and communicate with the hearing world without a lot of frustration.

Paula can. She fools a lot of people. Many people think she has no hearing loss at all. Many people think she is only moderately hard of hearing but in reality she has a profound loss. I think it is because she had a strong oral program while she was young.

Pauline Zamecki:

Perhaps that is true. Paula was in a strong oral program where she was taught to make the very most of her residual hearing. But as I look back, I feel this learning could have come about whether she had learned signs or not. If you teach both the maximum use of residual hearing and the use of signs at the same time, wouldn't you have the best of both worlds?

Richard Zamecki:

Maybe that would work. But from my experience, I still say: voice communication first; then, later, permit the use of sign. Otherwise, it is just too easy to rely on the use of signs and the voice will not be developed.

I feel that after Paula learned the use of signs, she just didn't use her voice as much with us, as well as with her friends.

Pauline Zamecki:

That too is true, but when she was put into this total communication environment her friends were no longer oral, they used signs. So she naturally went to the communication mode that her friends were using.

Richard Zamecki:

I'm just saying that if Paula had not first had orally based training, she would not be functioning as well as she is today.

Pauline Zamecki:

That may be true, but you have to remember that Paula was an exceptionally bright child. Not all the children in this situation are able to pick up language and speech as Paula was able to do.

Many oral programs will show you what their best students are able to do but they do not address the needs of the majority of the deaf population, those that are not able to function without the use of a sign language system.

I saw some oral students who never became oral. The program was a very strict oral program that did not permit any signs or gestures among the children. Unfortunately some of these kids simply didn't have the talent, the home environment, or the constant language reinforcement to make this work. So they went for years without any communication ability at all. They couldn't talk, they couldn't lip read, they couldn't write. Is that fair? I think that is scary.

Richard Zamecki:

Also, I believe that a teacher can make or break a child. I don't care if it is a oral program or a total communication program, if the teacher is not motivated, then get your child out of it and find a teacher who is truly motivated. Put your child with a teacher who cares, one who is really devoted. Find a teacher who doesn't care about the money (because it obviously isn't there), but one who really cares about teaching the children.

Ronald Kidder:

I can remember one instance quite clearly. We lived on a farm and Shannon had stepped on a nail. We rushed her to a hospital and the doctor had to probe to get the rust out of her foot.

We did not know sign language at the time and could not communicate with her. She was screaming and we could not explain to her that the doctor was really trying to help her. So for years every time she saw a doctor in a white coat, she would start crying. If we had been able to communicate with her at least she would have been able to understand what was happening. The physical pain would have been there, but at least she would have understood.

We see only positive results of a hard of hearing or deaf child learning sign language. There has got to be communication. If sign language is a better mode of communication, then the child has a right to that communication.

It is just like a Spanish child who speaks Spanish. Spanish is that child's first language. If the child wants to learn English and to communicate with English-speaking people, that's fine, but you don't take away communication in Spanish. The child simply becomes bilingual.

The deaf or hard of hearing child is the same. Learning signs does not detract from learning English. The child simply becomes bilingual.

Carolyn Lefever:

I think parents should learn sign language. Most of a child's language comes from the home. Teachers can really see the difference in children who come from homes with good communication.

A parent asks you whether he should send his child to a residential school or to a public school that has no previous experience with deaf children. How would you respond?

Joseph Livingston:

As I respond to this question I am thinking of a child who lives in a small town. I don't believe a school can set up a successful program for one child. The child needs to relate to other children and must have a comprehensive language program. If he is the only child in school that has a hearing loss, it is impossible to provide a good educational program.

I feel that I, as a parent, can not be my child's teacher. The child needs exposure to a variety of teachers to broaden his learning base. The child needs to learn from a math teacher, a science teacher, a reading teacher, etc.

If you have other children in the district with similar problems and you are able to convince the other parents to bring their children together in a small group, you might be able to set up a program. This assumes that you will find a teacher who can balance the needs of the child who is learning to read very slowly, verses the child who is picking it up very quickly.

Personally I would never send my child away from home. I might move to a city where a residential school is located, but I value the relationship I have with my children during the time they are not in school.

Cheryl Deconde Johnson:

If the child is profoundly deaf, I would probably suggest to the parents that they move. I hate the idea of breaking up the family, especially with very young children. Moving is probably not really necessary until the child is about three. Before then the programs are mostly home-based and could be done anywhere. But after the child reaches the age of three and is starting to branch out socially, he is going to need contacts with other deaf children.

I feel it is very important that the deaf child is not isolated. This can be a real problem in small communities. Even though the deaf child appears to function well, in reality, unless there are opportunities to communicate with other deaf children, the deaf child will experience a great deal of isolation.

I think that public day school programs can do a very nice job. Where I work, we have a large enough deaf population so that the children always have others they can communicate with on an equal basis.

There is a common argument made, that this type of program segregates the kids by centralizing them and that each child should attend her home school. Since the centralized program is within a regular K through 12 school there is the opportunity to integrate deaf, hard of hearing, and hearing students. Mainstreaming is important so long as it does not result in denying children access to information. Deafness is undoubtedly the most difficult handicap to mainstream effectively.

Communication is the backbone of the whole issue. Unless there are adequate numbers of peers for hearing impaired students to communicate with, they are segregated. Then you are dealing with a different type of isolation.

I really believe in centralizing deaf students. When the travel distance is excessive, I favor a regional day school concept where students are bused or live with other families during the week.

With the greater numbers you could have top-notch services within the regional centers. I would explore using existing residential schools as vocational training centers. Let the responsibility for primary academic training of the children be with the schools, at least until the children are sixteen or so. Then from ages sixteen to twenty-one, students could remain in their high school if they wanted to complete a college prep curriculum; or go to the residential style vocational training school that specialized in teaching independent living skills, vocational skills, technical skills, etc.

My response to the question of a day school versus a residential school, would be to consider the issues of maintaining the family unit and of finding the program with the best resources. Then find the solution that best fulfills both needs.

Andrew Nielsen:

I would ask a number of questions: What kind of a commitment are you willing to make? Are you willing to give up your Thursday night bowling league to learn to sign? Are you willing to take a lot of weekends to get your child out into the community? Are you willing to do all of this and more? If you are willing to commit yourself to these kinds of things, then keep your child with you at home. But if you are not willing to learn to communicate with your child, then send him to a residential school where he will not be isolated.

If you are in a small community which has no other deaf residents, I would recommend relocating. Find a community that has a deaf population that is large enough to support a good healthy program. Here in Greeley, we have about thirty-five deaf students and that is just barely large enough. You have got to have enough kids so that the child is able to select a friend.

You probably could get the child through the first or maybe even the third or fourth grades in a small town if the parents signed and you had an interpreter. But when puberty hits and the need to be with someone other than his parents becomes a factor, the child would need friends he could relate to.

Too many times the child in a small town becomes the "poor little deaf kid" and his lack of proper behavior is tolerated. He becomes more and more isolated. Hearing friends just do not fill the social and emotional needs of a child at this stage. I have seen many oral deaf students that can talk pretty well, and can function pretty well academically, but inside and socially they have some adjustment difficulties.

Donald Kitson:

I do not believe in residential schools. I do not believe children should be away from their parents or a home life. When children visit home during vacations, they become "homesick" for their friends at school. This is especially true if the children can not really communicate with their parents. The best, I believe, is a day school situation where the children are with their deaf classmates during the day and then are able to return home at night.

If the family was not able to move to such a day school situation, and the choice was between isolating the child in a hearing school or sending him to a residential school, I guess I would suggest a residential school.

Pam Pflueger:

Many students at the residential schools for the deaf develop a common bond. The students learn to accept their deafness because their peers are deaf, too. Socially, this is a plus. I have seen positive experiences from both private and public residential schools. Personally, I feel it would be best to move to a city where a day program or residential program is located. By being close to my child I would be able to guide her moral development. If moving is not possible, request that the local school provide a resource room teacher who is a trained teacher of the deaf.

My brother attended a special education school that was part of the public school system. All the children with disabilities in the entire school system were bussed to the same building. The children were then separated on the basis of disability. I felt this was difficult for the deaf students: neighborhood children assumed they were mentally retarded because they rode on the same bus and attended classes in the same school with mentally retarded students.

In junior high my brother was placed in a self-contained oral classroom in a regular public school. This was better, but I noticed there was a definite lack of group cohesiveness among the students compared to other programs for the deaf I had seen. The school did not actively encourage deaf students to participate in social activities with the hearing students, such as competitive sports. Parents have to be aware of whether the school setting is educating the whole child. Books are important but so is the social and emotional growth of the child.

Patty Pittroff Swain:

I would never have the child go to a public school where the staff had no previous experience teaching deaf children. The lack of knowledgeable support for the child would be catastrophic. There would be a lot of isolation and resulting withdrawal by the child. If this were the case, I would have to recommend the residential school.

My first choice would be for the family to move to a place that already had an established program for the deaf. The home environment could then be preserved for the child.

Richard Zamecki:

I would check out the residential school very closely before I took that option.

I would also want to check out the public school program. I think this would be better if there was a truly effective program for the deaf at that school.

I do feel that mixing deaf children with hearing children is a better influence for the deaf than having deaf children associate only with other deaf children. I feel the deaf students in a regular public school are able to respond to regular hearing students and that enriches them. You can't treat the deaf child in a different fashion than a hearing child.

Pauline Zamecki:

These are both bad choices! Let me say that to put a child in a program that has not already been established, is not education at all. Nobody there would be ready to handle the problems - not the teachers, not the other students. The child would be alone, learning to fear, being taunted, etc. If you send the child to a school where there has been no training, then you are wasting the child's time. For these reasons, I would say the residential school option would be the lesser of two evils. I really don't like that though, as you are leaving the teaching of morals, character, and behavior to somebody else.

Richard Zamecki:

This is true. I do not want somebody else bringing up my child.

Pauline Zamecki:

In response to Richard's feelings that you can't treat the deaf children differently than hearing children, I feel this is true up to a point. From our perspective, we are hearing people making judgments about the deaf culture. We say you should not be happy just associating with the deaf.

Maybe, though, that is exactly where the deaf want to be. They may be very much more comfortable with others who are like themselves. Is it right for hearing parents to say this is where we want you to be?

Richard Zamecki:

I think as far as schooling goes, if at all possible, make the special effort and relocate to a place that offers a good, already established program. I know it is hard to pick up and move and leave all your old friends and former job security, but in the long run it is a lot better for your child.

Sheila Kidder:

I don't like residential schools because they regiment the children. Kids come out of a residential school and don't know what to do unless someone tells them. On the other hand, the public school that has no previous experience is no help either.

The only answer to that question is move. We would demand that our child be in a good program where she has a chance to excel - but at the same time we would not send her away.

Socially, I see no problem staying in a neighborhood of only hearing children. Children adapt and make their own communication. Shannon and her hearing friends made up their own sign language. They each knew what the others were talking about.

At the same time, I feel that education is not just book learning. It is growing socially and emotionally as well as academically. It is imperative that your child not be isolated. If you educated a child in isolation, where the only thing the program gave her was academics, then that would be all she would learn.

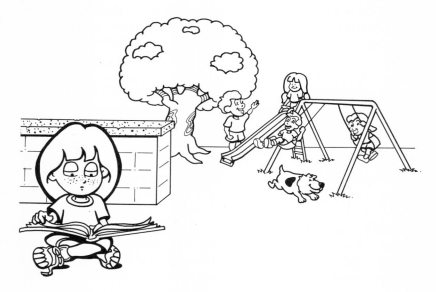

Since we lived in a neighborhood where there are no other deaf children, we felt it was important for Shannon to attend a school where there were other deaf students so she could grow socially and emotionally.

If the coach at the school does not want to be bothered with making the effort to communicate with a potential deaf player, what do you think the chances are of your child participating in sports? What are the chances of a girl being a cheerleader in a school where she is the only deaf student? How about the odds of becoming junior class president?

These opportunities are just not there for hearing impaired students in regular schools. There are limited opportunities for them to increase their self-esteem, confidence, and poise. You have to get them into programs where they can compete and be successful among their own peers.

A good day school for the deaf would be ideal. The family life remains intact, and the child is not the only deaf person at the school. Of course, the very big assumption here is that there is indeed a good academic program - a very big assumption in most instances!

Carolyn Lefever:

Personally, I think when parents send their kids away to residential school, the parents relinquish a lot: time with their children, opportunities to instill values, morals, religion, etc. On the other hand I have also seen kids in the public school who are essentially guinea pigs, and they suffer for it.

Educating a school and a community about deafness and starting a program from scratch would be too much. I would probably move to a community that had an established day program for the deaf.

What differences have you noticed between the social interactions of hard of hearing individuals and deaf individuals?

Joseph Livingston:

Many times the hard of hearing person is in a "never-never" land, not deaf and not hearing. The hard of hearing person feels isolated from the hearing world, and yet not a member of the deaf world.

I know of some hard of hearing individuals who function as though they were deaf. In an effort to join one of the two worlds, they decided to join the deaf world. Some of these individuals had good speech. They simply elected to turn it off and use only signs. These individuals were very reluctant to let the deaf world know that they were, in fact, hard of hearing. They wanted to be accepted as a part of the deaf world, and being hard of hearing was not acceptable.

A lot of people don't understand what hard of hearing means. Many people feel either you hear at a normal level or you are deaf, one or the other. The hard of hearing person knows there is a very large middle ground between these two extremes.

As far as social interactions, it is very much an individual thing. I would go so far as to say that social interactions are more a function of the individual than the amount of a hearing loss.

I have seen hard of hearing and deaf individuals function beautifully with hearing people, regardless of their own ability to hear. I have also seen hard of hearing and deaf people who could not function at all with hearing, other hard of hearing, or deaf people in social situations. It depends upon the individual.

Cheryl Deconde Johnson:

I think the hard of hearing person has a much greater disadvantage than the deaf person. When you are deaf, people accept that. They plan accordingly to communicate with you in whatever way necessary to get through the deafness.

Hard of hearing people usually use their hearing and speech well enough to get by. So the expectation is that they will function much like a normal hearing person. Most hard of hearing individuals frequently do things well enough to support this impression. The hard of hearing individual may constantly be in a state of stress, because he has to perform well enough to meet these expectations. This requires constant attending, listening, and keeping up with conversations, which are all very difficult.

Depending upon environmental factors, there will be times when the hard of hearing individual will function just fine and there are other times when that will be almost impossible. Hearing people don't understand this. They expect the hard of hearing person to function well at all times. They do not always show the patience for the hard of hearing individual that they show for the deaf individual.

For example, if an individual calls the name of a hard of hearing person and the person doesn't respond, the individual may think the person is stuck up. But if they know the person is deaf, the individual will understand why they did not respond. Hard of hearing individuals are really in a no-man's land. The deaf don't accept them because they can talk better and have more hearing. Hearing people hear most everything, and as a consequence, they are impatient and less understanding with those who don't hear as well as they do.

Andrew Nielsen:

The hard of hearing students have such a hard time. They develop their speech enough to give the appearance of functioning like hearing people.

Hearing people really don't understand. We don't even understand what it is like to have a temporary hearing loss.

The deaf child will not have a lot of the experiences the hard of hearing individual has. Again, the hard of hearing individual will hear just enough to get himself into stressful situations, but will not have enough hearing to easily get out of these same situations. The social pains and terrors are very real to the hard of hearing. Deaf individuals do not have to go through this.

I am surprised that we don't have more of our hard of hearing kids violently exploding against society. On the other hard, I have seen the hard of hearing kids do some things that are terribly cruel to their fellow students who are deaf. I suppose this is a reflection of some sort of pecking order, but that makes me angry.

My son, who is deaf, was at a gathering last week which was attended by a hard of hearing individual. Everyone was watching a captioned movie on TV. A commercial that wasn't captioned came on, and the hard of hearing person asked some of the deaf people to tell him what they thought the commercial was about. After they answered, he told them they were all really dumb, that the commercial was not about that at all.

This is an example of insensitivity that should not exist. Again, perhaps it is part of a pecking order. After you have been knocked down by the hearing world enough times, it feels kind of good to dish out some punishment yourself.

Now don't get me wrong, the deaf also have their problems in showing a lack of empathy for others. Many times the deaf have a hard time just understanding the concept of empathy.

For example, last week Joel and a group of his deaf friends were sitting at the dining table. After my wife announced that dinner was ready, I had to physically ask a deaf person to move over so that I could sit down at the dining table. This showed a complete lack of ordinary good manners. This probably results from the ways hearing people have treated this deaf person.

Hearing loss separates us from others. If you are not interacting with others, how do you develop the concept of otherness? "Me" is the only concept developed.

The difficulties of this can be reflected in those relationships between hard of hearing individuals and deaf individuals. These relationships can be very difficult to sustain because of the frequent occurrences of either real or imagined misunderstandings - and the different levels of empathy that have been developed by the parties involved.

Yita Harrison:

I have noticed that the hard of hearing, after they graduate, find that there are very few hard of hearing organizations, programs, or groups for them to socialize with. If they haven't done so already, they then learn sign language and end up joining deaf groups.

The same is true with many deaf individuals who were raised in oral programs. Most of them eventually learn signs and join deaf groups who sign. There is this constant integration of these two groups into the deaf world that sign. The reason for this is simple: communication. Without the communication of signs, these two groups feel isolated. The deaf world initially will not accept the hard of hearing individual who does not sign. The same is true for the oral deaf individual. After they learn sign language then the deaf world accepts them. Again, the reason is communication. Especially in a social situation, communication must be relatively easy and signs are the easiest way to achieve this.

I have seen deaf adults who do try to belong to the hearing world. In every case, success is very limited. One individual in particular comes to mind. This person refuses to accept her hearing loss. She has been successful in business, but she has no friends to socialize with.

Linda Hawbaker:

There are a lot of parts to this question. If you are talking about hard of hearing individuals who have not been around deaf people, then I think they act like their hearing peers. This is especially true in a school situation.

But if you have hard of hearing kids who have not been successful in the hearing environment and are then put into the hearing impaired environment, then I have seen a real difference. I have seen those kids overcompensating and overreacting, behaving as though they were deaf, even more than the deaf kids. I always thought that was rather interesting.

For example, I have seen the hard of hearing become totally immersed in an ASL type of language. I have also seen situations where a child with perfectly fine speech will then refuse to use it. I am not sure why this is. Perhaps it is a tremendous desire for acceptance by the deaf world. It could be that they are so comfortable in the deaf world that they want to emulate it completely. Then there is the possibility that in the company of deaf individuals, the hard of hearing person is no longer at the bottom of the social ladder, as opposed to when he is in the company of hearing individuals.

I think it depends upon the hard of hearing individual and the way he responds to the deaf world whether the deaf world accepts him or not. Bobby, our son who is deaf, really doesn't care if a person is deaf or hard of hearing.

I do think the hard of hearing individual has a more difficult time emotionally than the deaf individual. The deaf person doesn't hear anything. People know that and accept that.

Hearing people have a lot of frustration with those who do not hear well all the time; sometimes they seem to hear and at other times they don't. Those with normal hearing do not understand why there are these variances in the ability to hear. The hard of hearing individual has to deal with that animosity a lot more than the deaf individual.

Helga Simpson:

I know the hard of hearing individual has a very difficult time when he is involved in groups. These individuals are very frustrated because they have a hard time following the conversation. I think a lot of the hard of hearing prefer situations where there is just one other individual. It is easier for them to communicate in a one on one situation.

On the other hand, joining the deaf world and signing constantly is very tiring. The hard of hearing person who does not need to sign, and yet is frustrated in not being able to comfortably fit into many situations of the hearing world, has a very difficult time.

My daughter, Jenny, appears to be much happier when she is among other deaf people.

Pam Pflueger:

The hard of hearing individual appears to function in the hearing world socially, but he is often shy. At times he seems to be lost between the hearing world and the deaf world without an identity group to call his own. There are also many "oral" deaf individuals[14] who have longed for an identity group.

I know of three national organizations who have developed support services for hard of hearing and oral deaf individuals, Self Help for the Hard of Hearing (SHHH), which has 224 chapters across the country, was founded to form a support network for hard of hearing persons; the Alexander Graham Bell Association for the Deaf, which is active in promoting friendship for the hard of hearing and those who predominately use speech for communication; and the American Association of Late Deafened Adults.[15]

Patty Pittroff Swain:

The deaf have more of their own language and their own ways. There are social cliques. The hard of hearing also develop cliques. The reason for this is the different levels of communication.

Even within the deaf community, sub-cliques become established. Those that are more deaf tend to group with those who are also more deaf. Those that are less deaf tend to socialize with their peers who are also less deaf.

Pauline Zamecki:

When Paula has groups of friends at the house that consist of both hard of hearing and deaf people, I've noticed that the hard of hearing will at least attempt to communicate with the hearing people.

---

[14]These are severely hard of hearing or deaf individuals who received intensive auditory, speech, and speech reading training during their school years. They were not encouraged to learn or use sign language, but to rely upon their oral training skills for communication.

[15]See appendix for a complete listing of names, addresses and telephone numbers.

The deaf might as well be speaking German. They don't seem to see us. They do not make any effort to communicate with the hearing people present. If they don't have anybody to communicate with who knows signs, they just sit.

Sheila Kidder:

I think the deaf individual fairs better. The hearing impaired individual will strive to be a hearing person. The people who are hard of hearing tend to shun the deaf and try to be with hearing people. A lot of times this is for social status. Hard of hearing people do not necessarily have any true friends among hearing people, but they feel the hearing have a higher social status and they want to belong to that level.

The hearing world never really accepts them. The hard of hearing do not hear everything, and the hearing world doesn't want to take the time to repeat what is missed. The deaf are not concerned with that. Their attitude is "Well, here I am, like me or leave me."

I am not saying the deaf or hard of hearing person doesn't appreciate a hearing person who will take the time to learn their language, or make sure they understand a conversation.

It seems that the severely hard of hearing person will tend to join the deaf world and the moderately hard of hearing person will attempt to join the hearing world.

Even among the deaf, I feel there are distinctions. Those who were born deaf have an easier time socially than those who have lost their hearing at a later stage in life. Shannon, who was born deaf, has told us that there are only infrequent occasions when she really regrets being deaf. There are times she has actually said she felt lucky to be deaf because she doesn't have to put up with noise.

But people who have lost their hearing have lost a great deal. They have lost something they were accustomed to.

For that reason, I feel they have a harder time emotionally and socially. The first thing they think is, "Why me?"

Parents sometimes go through a similar struggle, a guilt battle that will have to be waged and dealt with. I can remember one person telling me that I was paying for my past sins by having a deaf daughter.

After the guilt and denial are dealt with, the best thing is to accept the situation and get on with your life. This is true for the parents as well as the individual who loses his hearing later in life. "Why?" is not important. How you deal with it is what is important.

To be candid, it took us, as parents, four to five years to fully accept Shannon's situation and become really comfortable with it. But we had nobody to talk with. It would have been a lot easier at the time if someone had told us to forget asking "Why?" because, whether or not there is an answer, the situation remains the same. Move on to doing what is best for the child.

Carolyn Lefever:

Deaf people are on the fringes of social interaction only when they are among hearing people who don't sign. Hard of hearing people are almost always on the fringes.

What differences have you noticed between the interactions of deaf children who have deaf parents, and the interactions of deaf children who have hearing parents?

Joseph Livingston:

I don't know of any really good studies that have been done comparing these two groups. I think children's development depends upon their parents and the quality of time they are able to spend with their children. I have seen deaf parents and deaf children that form wonderful family units. I have also seen deaf children with deaf parents that were not very well adjusted. I have seen hearing parents that have some really neat deaf kids, but I have also seen hearing parents with deaf children that were real disasters. I think it is the calibre of the parents that make the difference rather than the handicap itself. The handicap adds some factors, true, but if the parents work hard, these factors are not a barrier to a good family unit.

I think there is a need to be aware of the pitfalls of analyzing the handicap too much. Sometimes undue attention is given to the handicap and other common sense directions of parenting are forgotten. The handicap is only a part of the whole child.

Donald Kitson:

It is hard to say. Some deaf children of deaf parents have a better education because of a good home life. Frequently deaf children of hearing parents do not have the same quality of life at home. Their parents do not communicate as well or as frequently with their children.

I was very lucky. My parents are hearing. My mother was a school teacher. She and my father had a lot of patience with me. They constantly made the extra effort required to communicate with me.

I have also seen deaf parents who had very little education and their deaf children did very poorly in school. So having deaf parents does not, by itself, guarantee success in school or life. I think it depends upon the parents background, as well as on the amount and quality of time the parents are willing to spend with their child. This is true regardless of whether the parents are deaf or hearing.

Speaking for myself, I would want good parents. It would not make any difference to me if they were hearing or deaf. Good parents will give you a lot of motivation, love, sharing, and communicate with you.

I grew up with hearing parents that did not believe in sign language. They thought it would be a hindrance to my speech development. When I went off to college I learned sign language, and, at first, my parents were disappointed. Later, after they saw how much happier I was, they didn't mind.

While I was growing up I had to try to read their lips. If something was really important they would write it down. Even today they do not know sign language and we still frequently write things down.

The point is that even with this extreme barrier, my parents were good enough to take the time to communicate with me. They motivated me and were good parents in spite of my deafness. Good parents will not let deafness block the avenues of communication with their children, whether they use signs or not, and whether the parents are deaf or not.

Yita Harrison:
Years ago, deaf children who had deaf parents usually started out communicating at an earlier stage with their

parents. But today we have hearing parents who are actively learning sign language and communicating with their deaf children just as well as deaf parents. The communication lag has narrowed considerably. I must say, though, many times I will have a deaf student complain to me that his hearing parents don't understand what he is trying to say. I have never had a deaf child of deaf parents make that complaint.

Helga Simpson:

Just from a few observations I have made, I think the deaf children of deaf parents seem to be very bright. I think this is a result of the immediate language input they receive from their parents who have signed to them from day one.

Frequently the hearing parents will have to go through the steps of diagnosing the deafness, accepting the deafness, and then learning sign language before they are really able to get any language input to their deaf child. This creates a critical time lag where there is no language input. The deaf child of deaf parents does not have this time lag.

Pam Pflueger:

Deaf children who have deaf parents seem to accept themselves better than other deaf children. They are like their parents. They are accustomed to the same world as their parents. Their parents expose them to a visual language from the time of their birth.

Deaf children who have hearing parents have a much more difficult time communicating and knowing their family. Neither children nor parents ever really experience and understand the other's world. It takes a lot of work for both parties to feel psychologically and emotionally comfortable with each other. A lot will depend on how the parents work with their child.

Pauline Zamecki:

It seems to me that the deaf parent will have more patience to talk to, and deal with her deaf child. The hearing parent does not have the patience or the time.

Richard and I will talk about the social and other little interactions that we have gone though during the day. Paula does not get any of this because she can't hear it. We usually don't take the time to fill her in on what went on.

The deaf child with deaf parents will be able to pick up on these social conversations because of the constant use of signs. It is a lot easier for the deaf child in this case to feel part of a family.

If the hearing parents do not sign or only selectively sign, and do not make a real effort to include the child, he will feel he is only a visitor and not a part of the family unit.

For example, my other two hearing children know how Richard and I met, dated, and got married. Paula has no idea how we met or the courtship that we went though. We are her parents and she has no idea how we got together.

The other children have picked up on this over the years though informal conversations. For Paula to gather this bit of family history, we have to sit down and make an extra effort to consciously explain it to her.

It is the little things that she misses. She will wonder if there is something wrong with her as a teenager because she is scared about something. My other kids know this is not unusual, but does Paula? She has never heard all the small conversations that the other members of the family have had over the years. She has no idea that as a teenager, I was scared sometimes, too.

Even if the hearing parents learned sign language, there would still be the selective use of the sign language. Signing is slower than speech and more tiring, and hearing parents are going to talk with each other rather than sign. This would also be true between the hearing parents and the other hearing children, and between the hearing siblings themselves. The deaf child will miss out of a lot of the daily babble of the family.

It is good that the hearing parents learn and use sign language, but the family's communication will most likely be more accessible for a deaf child if he has deaf parents.

Any thoughts for deaf parents who have hearing children?

Joseph Livingston:

I have only known eight or nine families in which the parents are deaf and the children are hearing. I really think the parents must make a special effort to expand their children's horizons. Don't keep them in your world. Sometimes within a deaf community you find a relatively small operating world.

It is the same concept of living here in the mountains in a small town. Sometimes our children here in Basalt, Colorado don't see enough of what exists outside their immediate community. The world is a lot bigger than this nice little valley.

I think reading to young children is very important. For deaf parents this can be a major problem. Deaf parents should be aware that they can get recorded reading material. But you don't just turn the recorder on at the table and leave it. The parent needs to spend time with the child going over the story.

You want the child to build good speech. True, the child will be exposed to speech and language as she associates with other children, but every study I have seen emphasizes that early exposure is critical, and that comes from parents.

Andrew Nielsen:

Don't ever force your young hearing children to be your interpreters. If you are going to buy a car, do not expect your six year old son to negotiate the deal for you. Don't put them into that kind of situation. You will burn them out.

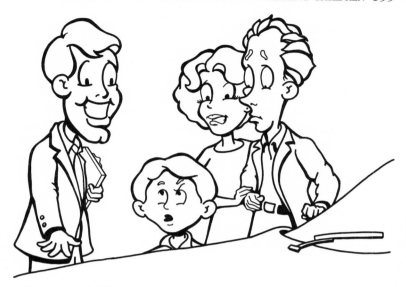

Let your children have access to other hearing kids. Realize that hearing children and their friends will play a lot of games with you. Kids will be kids.

The biggest complaint I have heard from hearing kids of deaf parents is the pressure they have felt by being forced to be their parents' interpreters, particularly at a young age. This is especially true when the situation involves large sums of money. Misunderstandings can lead to resentment between the parents and the children.

Frequently the relationship between hearing children and their deaf parents will go through several stages: first, not knowing your parents are different; then grasping the fact that your parents are different; later resenting this fact that your parents are different; gradually understanding that your parents love you and that they are pretty neat people; and finally wanting to tell the world about your parents. Of course, this is an evolutionary process that covers some twenty or more years of the child's development.

Paula Smith:

I believe there can be a real problem when deaf parents use their children as interpreters. Deaf parents must be careful not to become overly dependent upon their hearing children.

I have worked with professional interpreters who had to assume this role for their deaf parents at an early age. They shared with me their resentment of having to interpret for their parents. They felt overwhelmed by having to make decisions for their parents. This was especially true when the children were young.

They resented having to repeatedly explain their parents' deafness to others. They become tired of being the go-between for everything. There is a stage when this resentment can become so severe, that the children will not want to have anything to do with their parents. During adolescence this can lead to problems.

Donald Kitson:

I am a deaf parent with two hearing boys. Their mother is also deaf. Both boys have normal speech and no emotional problems.

Jason, my oldest boy, is thirteen and very shy. He does not want his friends to know that his father is deaf. He has passed this feeling on to his friends. They seem to be uncomfortable when they are with us.

Alvin, my youngest boy, is eleven and doesn't care one way or the other. His friends seem to be very comfortable when they are with us. Each of our children have responded differently to the fact that his parents are deaf.

When the boys were young, we taught them sign language. They were communicating with us before they were using their voices. Within a few months of their birth, both boys knew the sign for milk.

In regard to speech development, Jason seemed to have trouble saying his ts and ls. When he went into public school, he had special training to correct his speech. Now, his speech is fine. Alvin never had a problem with his speech development.

I remember one deaf parent I know who never used his voice. His young hearing son did not use his voice and always relied on sign language. When he was six years old and went into first grade, he had to make quite an adjustment to use his voice. He was quite successful and later became a famous legislator in the state of Florida. His skills as a orator were well known.

Speech development is not really that much of a problem. Hearing children will get their speech from bedtime stories on tape, records, television, radio, other children in the neighborhood and school.

Yita Harrison:

I am a deaf parent with three grown hearing daughters. If I could do it all over again there would be at least one thing I would change: I would not give my daughters as much responsibility as I did when they were young.

For example, when my oldest daughter, Karen, was three years old, she was already making business phone calls for me. One time an insurance man came to the door and wanted to meet the person who had called to arrange an appointment for me. He was shocked to find out that she was only three years old.

My children grew up with too much responsibility. Though they never seemed to resent this, I have seen other families in which the burden was too much for the children.

Today things are a lot better for deaf parents. They have access to TDDs[16] and relay services that allow us to communicate directly with people we need to be in touch with.

Also remember that there will be times your hearing children will be able to do more or experience more than you will. Do not hold that against your children. It is not your fault that you are deaf, and it is not their fault that they are hearing. Resentments and jealousies help no one.

---

[16]"TDD" stands for "Telecommunication Devices for the Deaf." It is a typewriter styled device that allows deaf and hard of hearing people to communicate over the telephone by typing messages to each other. Many businesses today have TDDs to serve their hearing impaired customers.

Does it make any difference if the deaf child in a family is the oldest child, the middle child, or the youngest child? Does it make any difference if the child is a boy or a girl?

Joseph Livingston:

It makes a difference primarily on how the family accepts the individual differences of the children. I think this depends on the individual families.

I don't think there is a real difference between families as to whether the deaf child is a boy or a girl. If the family unit is over-protective because the child is a girl or expects a macho personality because the child is a boy; I think these things will be present, in that particular family, regardless whether the child is deaf... but lets face it, birth order has an effect on all children.

Cheryl Deconde Johnson:

The situation that stands out for me is the one which the deaf child is the youngest. The youngest child tends to be treated as the baby of the family, if the child is also deaf, there is a tendency to do even more for him.

Andrew Nielsen:

I think the birth order has an effect on normal as well as deaf children. In our case, Joel is the oldest of our three children. He is deaf and the other two have normal hearing.

Joel structured the situation: because he was the oldest he set the tone. If the second child wanted to play with Joel, he had to interact with Joel via sign language. If the oldest child had been hearing and the second child was deaf, the oldest one would have found it a lot easier to just walk away. It is really not necessary to play with a younger sibling.

If the older child is deaf there is a danger of the parents unwittingly conveying the feeling that, because of his deafness, he is not as capable as the younger siblings. Then the oldest can run into some real problems with his self-concept.

We held the same standards for Joel as we did for any of the other children. Joel never got the feeling that he was any less capable than his brother or sister. We expected him to look after his younger brother and sister.

The biggest disadvantage about being the oldest and being deaf is that there is usually a longer period of time that elapses before the deafness is diagnosed. There is no previous child to compare this infant to.

I think in the near future, research is going to show that deaf girls have a better chance of developing language than deaf boys. I think the deafness is a bigger social handicap for a girl. Girls are more verbal, they tend to socialize more than boys. If a girl has a hard time socializing then she is really isolated.

Boys can go a long way on their physical skills. By participating in sports, boys have a way of raising their self-esteem. Joel gained a great deal from his ability to play football and participate in other sports.

Paula Smith:

I think if the deaf child is the oldest, he will get a lot more attention from the parents. His parents will have the highest expectations for him. This can be good or bad depending upon the manner in which it is done.

If the child is the youngest, frequently there will be a tendency to baby the child. The expectations will not be as high.

There is a tendency to see deaf girls in the traditional female role of pleasant homemakers. All they have to do is find the right boy, get married, and it is assumed that they will be taken care of. Deaf boys have a lot more pressure put on them. They are expected to go out, find a job, and compete with the hearing world.

This is changing, as it is with the hearing world, but the process has been delayed in the deaf world. The job opportunities for both deaf boys and deaf girls are opening up.

We need to encourage and foster the feeling among deaf girls that they can compete successfully in the job market. They should not rely on their deaf boyfriends to go on to further training and to provide for them.

Linda Hawbaker:

I am sure it makes a difference. It makes a difference with hearing children, so I am sure it makes a difference with a deaf sibling.

In most of the families I have known, the deaf child happens to be the oldest. I think it is pretty tough to be the oldest because not only is this first child a great experiment for the parents, but they are on totally unfamiliar ground when dealing with the deafness as well. Sometimes it is possible to get too involved in the hearing loss and not enough attention is paid to the parenting of the whole child.

As far as whether it makes a difference if the child is a boy or a girl, I think it is a matter of how the parents would react to the child regardless of the deafness.

Larry Hawbaker:

I think the easier route would be for the deaf child to be the youngest. The older siblings would pick up sign language very fast. To children, sign language is almost a game. So the youngest child would have a lot more sibling support in terms of language development and stimulation.

An oldest deaf child would, at least initially, have to rely upon the parents for all the sign language stimulation. Parents, because they are older, frequently find that learning sign language is more of a task than a game.

Helga Simpson:

That is not an easy question. I always felt my oldest son was jealous of my deaf daughter, Jennifer, who was a middle child. I believe he felt that I was giving her too much attention. I am sure this was true to an extent because of the time required for sign language and dealing with deafness. She did require my attention when she needed some help in communicating with the hearing world.

I think the best situation would be for the deaf child to be the youngest. The parents would have had the previous experiences of raising the earlier siblings and would know more about parenting. Instead of having to learn both parenting and dealing with deafness at one time, they would only have the deafness to contend with.

I think the parents will react in the same fashion whether their deaf child is a boy or a girl. It is an individual thing, and I think it would be the same whether the child is deaf or hearing.

Pam Pflueger:

I have heard that the deaf child who is the oldest often struggles the most because his parents are new parents, in addition to having to learn about deafness. The youngest also have their struggles. For example, older parents may not have the energy they had when they were younger, and raising a deaf child can require a lot more energy than raising a hearing child. For the youngest child in a single parent household, the struggles can be even more intense.

Patty Pittroff Swain:

I was in the middle, and I felt I was in the middle. You're not the oldest and you're not the baby. Who are you?

I did get a lot of attention, probably more than most middle children, because of my hearing problems. I know this created some resentment among my brothers and sisters.

My younger sister is only eleven months younger than I am. I always reacted to her as though she was my older sister, because she could hear and was much more tuned-in to everything that was going on. She was always ahead of me in meeting people and getting around.

As to whether there is a difference if the child is a boy or a girl, I don't think there is that much difference. If anything a deaf boy might be laughed at more than a deaf girl. A girl can hide her hearing aids underneath her hair easier than a boy, but there are those times a girl, too, will be laughed at.

I think it is much harder for a boy to try to fit into a social group, especially during the junior high and high school years. This is particularly true if the boy is trying to fit into a hearing group.

Richard Zamecki:

If you had a hearing child before you had a deaf child, it would be a lot easier. You would catch the deafness a lot sooner.

Pauline Zamecki:

True, but only for that reason. I feel that if you could catch the deafness soon enough, then it would be better if the oldest child was the deaf child. Then you would have more time available to spend with this child, than you would with younger children when your time is divided among the siblings. You could spend the maximum amount of time on language development and other communication skills with the hearing impaired child.

Richard Zamecki:

On the other hand, if the child was not oldest, then the older children would be there to help with their younger sibling. All the burden of communicating would not be resting solely upon the parents.

Pauline Zamecki:

Yes, but during the youngest years, the most important training years, the older children are too young to really help. It is only later, as the children become young adults that you see siblings really helping each other.

Paula, being the oldest, was quite assertive in setting up the pecking order with her younger siblings. She is very bright, perceptive, and sometimes quite stubborn. She thinks she is her younger siblings' boss.

Especially during the high school years, deafness did make a difference. Communication was not there between the children. I think the younger children tended to blame this on her deafness, which was partly the case. Another aspect was that they happened to have a bossy older sister.

Deaf or hearing, I don't think anyone should ever be a middle child. I was a middle child. You are in a never-never land of not getting the glory of the oldest and not receiving the attention of the baby of the family.

I think the first child has all the pressures from the parents. This is the first child, and maybe the last. All your dreams initially go into this child.

Richard Zamecki:

The younger one not only has to live up to the expectations of the parents, but also to the achievements of the older siblings. He has very little room for excuses because the older siblings have already accomplished this or that. What happens if he is never able to achieve those same standards?

Pauline Zamecki:

If the child is the youngest and the child is also deaf, there is a real danger. The child will be babied to start out with, and then if the child is deaf on top of that, the expectations can be so lowered that it is a real disservice to the child.

Actually, these same variables will be present in either hearing or deaf situations. The child you have happens to be deaf. All the other things that go into a child are there. Sibling rivalry, sibling caring, and sibling pecking order are all going to be there. The only thing that will be different is that there is the added challenge of deafness.

Because Paula was our first child, we treated her as we would have a hearing child and expected as much from her as from our other children. We expected her to mind, and when she didn't, she got spanked. If you don't have discipline, you will shortly have a tyrant.

It is the same with hearing kids. You have to remember all kids will test you to see what they can get away with. We simply treated Paula and her hearing siblings in the same fashion. No excuse was made for her deafness. Whether she was the oldest or deaf didn't make any difference.

If you don't discipline the child because you say the child doesn't understand, you are fooling yourself. Shortly the child will pick up on this and play on it. You are in for some real problems. And, remember the name of the game is not to physically hurt the child, it is to get the child's attention. Sometimes that requires a spanking, but usually a severe look with good eye contact will be more than sufficient. And when a spanking is necessary, the hand is quite enough. I feel that once you resort to something like a paddle, you have lost the point of spanking.

As far as a deaf girl versus a deaf boy, the boy has a lot more to adjust to. A deaf girl can always get married. There are not the expectations placed on her to establish a career that will support a family.

A deaf boy sometimes has to contend with an attitude that says, "Well, you are limited to what they can teach you in vocational school. In anything more than that, you are probably going to be a failure."

Richard Zamecki:

I think parents need to give that extra effort to help the boy to overcome this. They need to boost him in his ability to achieve what he wants.

Sheila Kidder:

We have a saying in our house: "We learned on the first three, the last three have it easy." On your oldest child, you learn. It is hardest for this child. You expect more of this child.

The baby is treated with special care because this is the last one and you know it. The middle one is just there.

To be the youngest and deaf would be too special. That would be a dangerous combination of potential over-protection. I think the best position for a deaf child would be that of a middle child. The parents would have had a chance to learn a little on the oldest, without the danger of doting that could occur if the deaf child was the youngest.

Socially, I think boys have a lot more peer pressure to contend with than girls. If the boys don't have a stable home, or someone they can rely on, then there is a real danger for them. I think, vocationally, boys and girls get the same treatment. If you are going to successfully deal with the hearing world, you are going to have to make an effort.

Have you noticed a difference between mothers and fathers in accepting the fact that one of their offspring is deaf or hard of hearing? What do you think the reasons are for any differences?

Cheryl Deconde Johnson:

I think that this depends on the family. In some families, the mothers are going to accept the situation more easily than the fathers, and in other families it is the other way around. Some parents accept things very readily and move on. Other parents do not. Those parents who never accept their child's deafness are very frustrated people. Their child is never what they wanted him to be.

Unfortunately the children sense this. They feel they can never meet their parents' expectations. They, in turn, become very frustrated. Parents need to help their children develop as fully as possible without the weight of unrealistic expectations.

Acceptance usually comes in stages. Frequently parents will accept some limitations, especially those present at the time. As the child grows older additional problems become evident. With each one another acceptance is made. In this way parents gradually understand and accept the limitations of their child.

Here in Greeley, children and parents are able to mingle and see each other at all ages. I think it is good for preschoolers to see other deaf or hard of hearing children who are ten or fifteen years old. Young children may not be able to express what they see, but they can begin to understand what is ahead in five years or more. The security of knowing that there is a future before them is very comforting.

It is also very good for the parents of preschoolers to see the older children. They can become more familiar and comfortable with what lies ahead for their children. Much of the fear of the unknown is then eliminated.

Andrew Nielsen:

Acceptance can be difficult for different reasons. Mothers are eons ahead of fathers. It seems to me that men have a much more difficult time comprehending that something is wrong with a child. A father will frequently judge a baby by its looks. You can't see this handicap, so it is difficult to believe there is something wrong. "But, my son looks so normal!", fathers will say.

Women generally have better fine motor skills. Men seem to have superior gross motor skills. Some men have a harder time learning to sign. My wife picks up signs a lot faster than I do.

A man will have more concern about his son's or daughter's status within a group. He also will have more of a tendency to walk away from the problem. Part of this tendency goes back to Biblical times and the attitudes established then. Adam had to be concerned with physically providing for the family. Eve's concern was to take care of the emotional needs of the family. The ramifications of this approach are still with us. The father buys the hearing aid and his job is done. The mother has this on-going responsibility for the affection and emotional support of the child. The mother takes the time to learn how to sign, but the father doesn't need to (or didn't have the time because he was too busy earning the money to pay for the hearing aid).

On the other hand, some women will use a handicapped child as a means to martyrdom. That girl who was not the homecoming queen is now special because she has a handicapped child.

Paula Smith:

It is hard to generalize. I think it depends upon the individual parents. How secure do they feel in themselves and with each other?

I think it is sometimes harder for the mother to accept the fact that the child is deaf or hard of hearing. The mother often wants to protect the child from any negative situations that may arise. Frequently, the mother will be more emotional in the support of the child, and the father will be more objective.

The father looks at the child more from an economic viewpoint. What will the child do to support himself in the future? What financial burdens are there going to be?

The mother may feel guilty, feeling responsible for doing something during her pregnancy that caused her child's deafness. This most likely is not the case, and she needs to put this dragon to rest.

I would strongly encourage parents to seek support from other parents or a counselor who is familiar with deafness so they can talk about things. This can help put fears and anxieties to rest.

Donald Kitson:

I think a mother will accept it easier than the father. This causes a lot of divorces. Fathers are frequently embarrassed that a family member is handicapped. They are embarrassed to tell their co-workers that they are the father of a handicapped child. They feel they can not hold up the image of a good life at home.

My father loved my mother so much that he loved his wife's children, regardless of their condition. Not many fathers are like that today.

Yita Harrison:

The mother is more likely to accept the handicap. The father imagines himself as the perfect person in the family. Nothing can be wrong that comes from him. "The person born from me is perfect. If there is an imperfection, it is my wife's fault."

This attitude results in the father leaving the home. He leaves his wife to deal with the deaf child. He buries himself in his work. He comes home afterward, reads the paper, and goes to bed. He doesn't want to be burdened with the child or his problems. In extreme cases, he avoids the whole situation by getting a divorce.

Pam Pflueger:

I think in most families there tends to be one parent who is the key communicator within the family. It can be either the mother or the father, but both need to understand what is involved in raising a deaf child.

I think in most situations during the time the child is very young the mother usually spends more time with the child than the father. The mother will therefore receive an earlier and more intensive education as to the special needs of her deaf child. It is she who will be instructing and interacting with the child during the majority of her waking hours. She really has no choice and accepts her role as mother/educator.

The father has less exposure to the child, and it may take longer for him to understand the avenues that need to be traveled, the situations that need to be experienced, and the accomplishments that can be achieved.

Ideally both parents will contribute in their own way to the education of their child. My mother took a more active role in the academic aspects, and my father reinforced the academics with daily speech and auditory training activities.

When my mother passed away my father had to assume total responsibility. This was a tremendous challenge and adjustment. He had to teach himself how to become an educator and to keep providing educational stimulation to my brother.

Pauline Zamecki:

The mother is more involved in raising the children. The father is away working. It is the mother's job to raise the children. Frequently there is no choice. Somebody has to work to earn money, and somebody has to raise the children.

When the father comes home from work he is tired. Home is the place where he should be able to relax, not start another part-time job. If the wife is not working outside of the home, then this is her job, dealing with the children.

Frequently the mother has no choice: she must accept the child handicap and all. The father has a choice: to escape into his job, or even get a divorce. If a divorce occurs the child usually goes with the mother, again, handicap and all.

Richard Zamecki:

I tried to excel in my job so that I could get the things for Paula that she needed. I do not feel that Paula's being deaf put any more pressure on my marriage. I gave up a few things. I became more responsible a little faster. I felt we needed the money. I didn't resent Paula for that: Paula didn't choose to be deaf.

After we found out that she was deaf, we just went from there. No denial, just what do we need to do, and let's get on with it.

Pauline Zamecki:

In life there is not always somebody to blame for something. It is just life. Finding fault or denial of the situation serves no purpose. Take care of the situation and go on from there.

Ronald Kidder:

I have seen it both ways. Sometimes mothers will accept the deafness, and fathers will deny it. Other times, the father accepts the deafness, and the mother denies it.

In the case of the fathers, I think frequently fathers can not accept that they are associated with a handicapped child because they feel it changes their social status.

Sheila Kidder:

I have seen the same in mothers.

Ronald Kidder:

I have seen some parents blame all the family's problems on the loss of hearing.

Sheila Kidder:

I think the problems I have seen with families that have deaf children are due more to a lack of communication between the parents themselves, rather than the fact that a child came along who was deaf or hard of hearing.

If the communication was there, they would have worked together and helped each other accept it. Without the communication, they go their separate ways for whatever reason.

Ronald Kidder:

Sometimes this can be as a result of misplaced guilt. Either the person wrongfully assumes the guilt of having a deaf child or puts it on the other parent.

Sheila Kidder:

For example, my father has two deaf cousins. When Shannon was born, he felt it was all his fault that Shannon was deaf! Come on, get real! Shannon was deaf and it could have been for any number of a thousand reasons. Who cares? Let's get on with finding out what is best for her.

If anything, Shannon brought us closer together. She has so much affection. The deaf are more physical in their demonstrations of affection. They do not hide it. They show you how to love. By having her I think she taught us to be more aware of our other children's needs. She made the family unit stronger.

What is the best way for hearing parents to communicate with their deaf child?

Joseph Livingston:

I don't think there is a "best way." I think it depends upon the parents, upon the children, the degree of hearing loss, their backgrounds, etc.

I know of some profoundly deaf individuals with bilateral 90 db losses who function very well auditorially and through speech. I don't believe they would be better off if they signed. On the other hand, I don't believe they would be worse off either.

I believe in disciplining the hearing impaired child with the same standards as a hearing child. You have to make sure, though, that you have the child's visual attention.

It is also a lot more tiring to discipline a hearing impaired child, especially if you are using sign language as your primary means of communication. You are going to have to get up out of your comfortable chair, go over, and visually get your message across.

Discipline requires a lot of love, understanding, and patience. You do not have to be harsh with a deaf child - or with a hearing child. With all children you first must have their attention, and second, you must make sure they understand why they are being disciplined.

A lot of times you may be trying to correct or change a pattern of behavior that they don't know is a problem. So you need to do it with "kid gloves."

Deaf kids many times learn how to use the "I don't understand" look very effectively. As a parent you must learn to differentiate those times when your child does indeed know what is expected of him, from other times when he genuinely does not understand.

If the child is so angry, that he turns away from me and refuses to look at me while I am trying to address him, I back off. My attempts to discuss the problem with him at this time would be largely a wasted effort. So I ask him to sit down and cool off for a while. Then we talk things over.

Cheryl Deconde Johnson:

For the deaf child, I think the best way is a combination of signed and vocal communication: any way that will allow meaning to be transferred between the individuals involved.

The critical element when you discipline a deaf child, or any child for that matter, is that they understand why they are being disciplined. To do this you have to be able to communicate with your child.

With hard of hearing children, you have to make the extra effort to make sure they understand the whole message. Frequently they only understand a part of the message, or misunderstand the whole message and act upon that.

What I see frequently, and it is unfortunate, is that many parents will discipline their children, but will not take the time to explain why because they do not know enough sign language. We need to lay out actions and consequences to the child: this is what happened, this is what you did, this is why it is not acceptable, and these are the consequences. We need to also let the child explain the circumstances to us. This takes some good communication skills, particularly when it involves sign language.

Andrew Nielsen:

The first rule is honesty. The second is communication: it all starts with a hug.

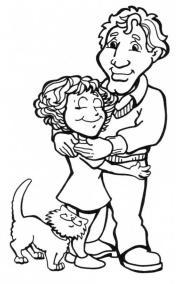

If I had to do it all over again, the things I would do differently! If only we had known that Joel was deaf when he was six months old, all the extra-sensory inputs we would have added...

· Everything that aids in communication and understanding should be used: verbal, signs, finger-spelling - everything that you can use that helps, use it.

Pam Pflueger:

Whatever method you use, be aware that your deaf child will initially not be on your language level. You will need to simplify your vocabulary and sentence structure to ensure your child really understands. When you introduce new vocabulary, you will need to compare and contrast it with established terms.

Always test your child to make sure. Do not accept a simple nod of the head. Many times people will nod their heads simply to get out of the situation, even though they don't really comprehend what is being discussed. Do not wait for your child to ask questions, because the incidental learning that occurs in a hearing child, does not happen with a deaf child.

Memorizing words does not mean understanding them, and if your child doesn't understand them, what meaning do they have for him? For example, my brother memorized and orally recited daily prayers at meal times. The abstract words and concepts of the prayers were difficult. At first he did not understand what these words meant and had a difficult time saying them. As my father explained the words to him they became more meaningful.

You also need to be flexible with your daily schedule and habits. A hearing impaired student I know was expected to sit through church services that were not interpreted. Her parents could not understand why she was daydreaming or even falling asleep. There was an interpreted service of the same denomination available in the town, but the location and time were not as convenient, so this student endured an unintelligible service and had many opportunities for daydreaming.

Initially some members of my family spoke loudly to my brother and expected him to respond appropriately. They did not realize that he was simply attending to a loud sound and couldn't really understand the words.

Nor did they understand the limitations of a hearing aid: speaking louder sometimes actually made it more difficult for my brother to understand. If your child is wearing a hearing aid, make sure you are aware of the background noise in the room. Remember that the hearing aid is going to magnify all sounds. If you are trying to communicate or discipline your child orally, then the noise of the TV or the dishwasher will only hinder your efforts.

My father loved to whistle. Everybody in the family enjoyed his melodies except my brother. The whistling really had a negative effect on him because the hearing aid amplified the sound to an uncomfortable level. It took a real effort on my father's part to stop whistling whenever my brother was in the room.

Richard Zamecki:

Well, if things really became difficult, we would write down what we wanted to say. Of course, this was possible only after Paula had learned to read. We were able to do this when she was four years old.

Pauline Zamecki:

I would say communicate with your deaf child in any way you can. Use anything. Make him feel that you care enough to try. However, lip reading alone is quite difficult.

Initially, we labeled everything in our house: chair, table, bed, etc. Things that hearing kids pick up naturally from hearing words and sentences, need to be taught to a deaf child.

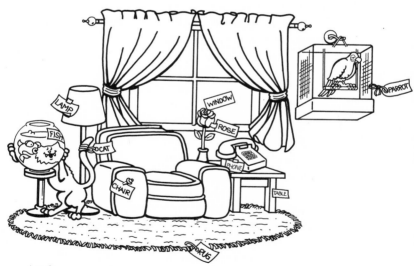

And you can't expect the school to do it all. At school, they are teaching certain things. But when your child comes home, you have to continue with that education with those things that the school doesn't get into.

Whenever I would move into a new neighborhood, I would frequently become involved with the neighborhood activities. I would make it a point to let the kids know that Paula was deaf, and allow them to become comfortable with that. I would show them Paula's hearing aid and let them listen to it. This would remove the mystery of the hearing aid from her hearing neighborhood friends. This helped her gain acceptance from the other kids in the neighborhood.

Ronald Kidder:

Learn sign language! Before we learned sign language, it was a constant battle. Getting Shannon dressed in the morning resembled a wrestling match. Then she would go to school and battle the teachers. The whole day seemed to be one constant battle.

After we learned sign language and Shannon learned sign language, it was a whole different ball game...What a difference!

I think it is so sad to see high school kids who still are not able to communicate with their parents, because their parents have not learned to use sign language.

Sheila Kidder:

Yes, I agree. And the parents will say, "No way, I am not going to learn sign language. She can talk!"

Well, come on. Give me a break. That may be workable to some extent, but speaking requires so much effort and leads to so much frustration on the kid's part that I question how much communication is really going on.

Shannon's initial program was oral. The staff did not accept sign language. They would slap the hands of the children if they attempted to use signs. So we moved 2,000 miles to a program that accepted signs. By using both signs and verbal communication, we were able to get on with Shannon's education.

What are your thoughts on the use of hearing aids?

Cheryl Deconde Johnson:

My bias is very pro hearing aids. When they are introduced with very young children around six months of age, they become a part of the child.

We have a very strict orientation program. The parents are always in control of the policy: that hearing aids are always worn. If that is established at the very beginning, then generally there is no adjustment problem. The kids will wear the hearing aids and put them on just as they get dressed in the morning.

The technology has improved greatly, so we are doing a better job in matching the loss with the type of aid. Frequently with the very young we are using a behind-the-ear type of hearing aid. Of course, with a profound loss the benefit is not going to be as great as it will be for a moderate loss.

I think one of our biggest weaknesses is that we are not working hard enough to develop auditory skills in children. We spend so much time in school with "information input." The school day is just not long enough for all the things that need to be done. We need to set aside a period in which we can do the direct communication therapy required to enhance the aural and oral communication skills of the children. We have to rely on parents to cover a lot. Schools can't do it all. We try to teach our parents to reinforce the speech, to make the effort to communicate with their child, to work with the hearing aids, etc.

Probably the only kids for whom I would not recommend hearing aids at a young age are those kids who have no cochlea at all. If there are no nerves to stimulate or amplify, then why bother?

As kids get older, there will be periods of time that they do not want to wear the aids. I think it is up to the parents and the school to insist that the aids be worn.

I know the kids say they sound awful and that they are not getting enough benefit from them. I know our kids with a profound hearing loss rely very heavily upon signs for input in instruction. They don't use their hearing very efficiently. In spite of all of this, I think they should be worn.

Up to the age of fourteen to sixteen the children should be told to wear their aids. After that, they are old enough to begin to make their own decisions in this matter. Kids go through many stages in puberty, and parents may feel that they should deal with matters more important than wearing a hearing aid.

I think the home is the key to the education of the child. Modeling is very important, especially with hearing impaired children.

Children, who see their parents actively involved in their education, such as attending school functions, talking with teachers, and following up on school education at home, learn that school is important. Parents are the key. Schools can't do in six hours all the things that parents want them to do. There is a need to establish a partnership between the school and the parents.

Andrew Nielsen:

You owe it to your child to give them as much input as possible. That means using the hearing aid. But when they get to be fourteen to sixteen years old, they should be allowed to make the decision as to whether to continue to use the aid or not.

"Does that hearing aid do enough for me to make up for the stares I get from others?"

"Does it benefit me enough to make up for the fact that I will be looked at differently?"

Yita Harrison:

I think back to a friend of mine. He used to be the Executive Secretary of the National Association of the Deaf. He wrote a paper that impressed me. He talked about both hearing aids and speech therapy at the same time. He said: when a deaf child is very small, he is forced to use hearing aids and develop his speech. As the child grows up even more emphasis is placed on hearing aids, speech, and language. Finally, as an adult, he has had enough, and decides not to use the hearing aid at all.

The pressure to use the aid and develop speech is constant for the deaf child. So when they become old enough to have a say in the matter, they toss out the pressure and its most obvious symbol: the hearing aid.

Helga Simpson:

With very young children, I would encourage the use of the hearing aid. Very young children accept it more readily, and if it helps, they will continue to use it.

As they become teenagers, if they say it is a distraction, it bothers them, or they don't like it for reasons of appearance, I would let them make up their own minds. Teenagers are very sensitive.

For adults, I would encourage them to use their aids, but it is up to them. If they say it is not really benefiting them, then why force the issue?

Pam Pflueger:

Though hearing aids will not correct hearing like glasses correct vision, they can assist in the child's learning and language development depending upon the severity of the loss. Some people like their hearing aids very much. When my brother first received his hearing aid it was like someone had turned on the lights in a dark room. You could see the reaction in his eyes. He did not want to take his aid off to go to sleep. Even today if his hearing aid battery dies, he wants an immediate replacement. He wants the auditory stimulation he gets wearing his hearing aid.

In the classroom I expected my students to wear their hearing aids and attempt to use their residual hearing as much as possible. As an elementary teacher I felt this was important.

Some teenagers are embarrassed about wearing hearing aids. If this is the case, show them positive role models that use hearing aids. Jennifer Parker representing the state of Washington in the 1989 Miss America Pageant is hearing impaired and was obviously wearing her hearing aid on television during all her performances.

Hearing aids do not always benefit the user because of the type of hearing loss. Ultimately, each individual must be allowed to decide whether or not to use the hearing aid.

Patty Pittroff Swain:

I would definitely use hearing aids with the very young, but I would caution people to make sure they are not too powerful. There are programs that encourage the use of a lot of power, and I feel that can be abused. If the person is profoundly deaf to where the hearing is not really being stimulated, and the aid is shaking the head with vibrations, where is the benefit? Who would be comfortable with that?

Many headaches and other trauma can result from this over-amplification.

Teenagers should wear their aids. I know they don't want to because of appearance. But if they don't, they could appear dumb. And nobody wants to appear deaf and dumb.

Whenever I am with people I always tell them I am hard of hearing. Otherwise they will think I am ignoring them when I don't respond, or they might think I am stupid.

I get so tired of trying to listen to people, I frequently just nod my head when they are talking to me. I don't understand what they are saying, but it is easier. That can be very embarrassing if your nodding and smiling is not an appropriate response to the conversation being directed towards you!

Richard Zamecki:

I think it is a good idea. Babies need to have the reinforcement of their own cooing. This can only help to encourage their own speech development. Once they quit, it is very hard to get speech development started again.

Pauline Zamecki:

I was always told it is best to encourage the use of the residual hearing. You can't use it if you don't know you have it. You have to keep fine-tuning it. You have to keep using it again and again, so over time auditory inputs become meaningful.

One of my greatest thrills was when Paula was eight. I yelled up the stairs to her to come to dinner. She responded, "OK, in a minute!" Using her residual hearing, she was able to respond to the meaning of my sentence. Without the training she would not have been able to respond as she did.

Richard Zamecki:

It is also, not only the word itself, it is how it is said, and the expression on your face when the word is being spoken, that give it meaning.

Pauline Zamecki:

Paula is completely tuned-out without her hearing aid. She knows it. She is never without her hearing aid. She enjoys the self-sufficiency that the hearing aid gives her.

Richard Zamecki:

True, but there were times when she rejected the aid. There were times she would take it out and throw it on the ground. We just had to keep encouraging her to put it back on again and again. We tried to make it a part of her. I think that helped. Now, as an adult, she wants it on all the time. She doesn't want to miss anything.

Pauline Zamecki:

With older people, there is a tremendous resistance to the use of hearing aids. They don't want to accept getting older. A lot of it is pride.

Older people and hard of hearing people should realize the other side also: a hearing loss puts a lot of pressure on the hearing people around them. The constant need to repeat words, and phrases, and raising your voice is tiring.

The hearing aid can help tremendously in allowing the older person not to look stupid in the company of others. He or she can respond in a more appropriate fashion.

Ronald Kidder:

Hearing aids will teach a child to start listening.

We are using behind-the-ear and all-in-the-ear hearing aids with babies. This gets them started.

Sheila Kidder:

The main problem we have with hearing aids is the misconception about them. People think they are just going to stick them in the ear, the hearing will be restored, and everything will be wonderful. That is not the case.

It is a learning process that is sometimes tedious. We put our people on a special schedule. They are only allowed to wear hearing aids for certain periods to help them get used to the aid. At first the brain will rebel at the added noises.

It is imperative that you have a hearing aid dispenser who will work with you, who will advise you, who will answer the telephone, who will address your questions to help you through that learning period. You cannot learn to use the aid in thirty days. An ideal schedule would require three to six months.

Ronald Kidder:

The sooner you get the hearing aid on a child, the fewer adjustment problems you will have to fight. There are fewer stigma problems of acceptance that we see with older children and adults.

With senior citizens, the attention span is sometimes very short. So the training during the learning/adjustment period is prolonged. Learning to use the hearing aid sometimes takes a lot of time for older patients.

They also have a very difficult time isolating sounds. The environment of a noisy cafeteria or nursing home makes it very hard for them.

Hearing aids are not for everybody. There are four stages one must work with to successfully use these devices. First, the person must accept the fact of the loss and seek help. Many times older people buy a hearing aid because the spouse or the family wants them to get one. So they put out a lot of money, and the aid promptly goes into the dresser drawer and that is where it stays. The three other stages are desire, effort, and patience.

Carolyn Lefever:
If there is usable residual hearing, it should be aided. From the teacher's point of view, it is always easier to teach a youngster who has learned to use his residual hearing effectively.

However, as an adult user of hearing aids, I don't like them: they are very uncomfortable!

*A student or child of yours refuses to wear her hearing aid.
What would you do?*

Joseph Livingston:

At some point you have to give the individual control over making the decisions for his destiny. I am reminded of an individual I know. When he wore his hearing aid, he functioned very well as a hard of hearing person. However, he elected to function as a deaf person and so he did not wear his aid. He was twenty-five years old and he wanted to be "deaf,"...and I guess that is his choice.

If the person is in junior high or high school, I would talk to him about it. But at some point you have to let the individual make his own decisions. Is he receiving enough benefit from wearing that hearing aid to warrant using it?

I wear my glasses because I can see better with them. If I did not receive sufficient benefit, I would not wear them - and I would resent someone telling me I must wear them. I can determine for myself as to whether the so-called benefits warrant their use.

I suspect that we really don't do enough in the individual fitting of the hearing aids. If a child seems to be rejecting the aid, then we need to find out why. Some aids are very powerful and need to be tailored to the specific individual. They need filters and boost-limiters to address the precise hearing loss of that individual.

This fitting is sometimes a long tedious process. It requires lots of time. Frequently people do not want to pay for that much time. If people were willing to pay for it, we could do a lot more true custom fitting of hearing aids.

Cheryl Deconde Johnson:

I think it is just like wearing glasses. If the child is really benefiting from them, they will wear them everyday. When the benefit is marginal then it is more difficult to make children wear them. As the hearing loss enters the profound range, a lot of individuals elect not to wear their aids. There are also students that have a difficult time dealing with anything that makes them different when they enter puberty.

I feel the kids that can benefit from the use of hearing aids should be encouraged to continue in their use. Perhaps some counseling could help them through adolescence.

Andrew Nielsen:

Well, I don't think there is going to be a right or wrong answer to this. You need to sit down with the child and find out exactly why he is rejecting the aid. Does the aid hurt his ears? Is it because the other kids are laughing at him?

If it is a situation of a hard of hearing child in a hearing environment, then I would sit down with him, and ask him if he would like me to address the class. If his classmates are ten years old, they may be laughing at him because they don't understand.

Now, let's imagine it is the deaf students who are teasing the hard of hearing student because he is wearing his hearing aid. That happens a lot. The taunt, "You trying to be hearing?", can be very painful.

Every case is unique. Individual counseling is required to deal with these situations. You talk with the child. You talk with the parents as to what their child is going through. The bottom line is: does the hearing aid help? If the child says it does, you tell him to toughen up to the occasional teasing: "If it benefits you, then it is your right to wear it. After a while the kids will accept it as a part of you, and will stop teasing you when they can no longer get a response."

A similar situation occurs with our deaf students sometimes. If they are profoundly deaf and have very limited understandable speech, they have to confront reality and think how they are going to communicate with the hearing world.

We encourage them to get into the habit of carrying a pen and notebook pad. Initially we get a lot of resistance from some of the students. We respond, "OK, you go and order lunch today at the restaurant." Or, "You are stopped by the police, how are you going to communicate - with sign language?" Better start making it a habit to have that pen and small notebook on hand.

Ronald Kidder:

I am reminded of a client of ours who is eighteen now. When we first worked with her, she was very excited because she could now hear noises that she couldn't hear before.

When she went to school she was mainstreamed. She was sixteen at this time. Her friends started to make fun of her. They would tell her she didn't have to wear her hearing aid, that she could hear just fine without it. Finally, the peer pressure was so intense she decided she didn't want to wear her aid.

Peer pressure is one of the hardest things for kids to face. Even deaf kids face a lot of this. Most deaf kids will wear just one hearing aid. They do not want to wear two because most of their peers only wear one. When they wear two hearing aids, the kids make fun of them.

Shannon has gone through stages of not wanting to wear her hearing aids. She has thrown them away, she has given them away, she has "lost" them.

Sheila Kidder:

Oh yes, I found one hearing aid that had been "lost" for two years. It had been buried underneath a plant. I was pulling up the plant to re-pot it and there was the aid!

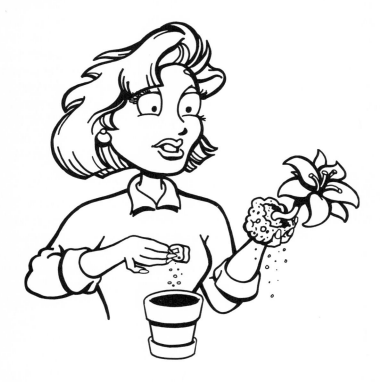

That aid was "lost" when Shannon was about fourteen years old. I made her do without her aids for an entire summer. I told her they were just too expensive, and she was just going to have to live without them for a while. So she went for three months without any sound. She found out that she didn't like that very much. From that time on she has taken very good care of her aids.

Ronald Kidder:

Understand that when a severely hearing impaired child first gets a hearing aid, all they hear is noise. When they have been previously accustomed to a quiet world, this rush of noise can be very unsettling.

Shannon has said to us many times she is happy to be deaf, so that she does not have to suffer all the distractions that noise seems to bring. When she really wants to concentrate on something she will take her hearing aid off. This is OK. There are times when quiet is just fine.

You should never force any child to wear a hearing aid. He has to be convinced himself that the benefits are worth the effort.

I have had situations arise where the husband and his wife would come in and want to buy a hearing aid for the husband. The husband would say that he was not really interested in wearing the aid, but was going to buy one so that his wife would shut up and stop nagging him about wearing one. I tell the couple that I do not at this time really want to sell them the aid. When the husband wants to buy and wear the aid on his own, then I will be happy to help him.

What are your thoughts on the usefulness of formal speech reading training?

Joseph Livingston:
I've seen it done, but I have never seen a real scientific analysis of it. I have always felt it was more of an art than a science. If it is an art, then there are certain things an instructor can point out to an individual. But I think it is very difficult to teach lip reading to someone who does not have an underlying skill for it.

I feel the instruction spent on teaching people how to take advantage of lip reading clues are worthwhile, but I don't think you can take anyone and make him an excellent lip reader. It is a lot like painting. Just because you teach a person some painting techniques doesn't mean you will make that person a good painter.

This is a little off the point, but as far as educational programs go, I think the overriding factor is the individual child. The overall rate of learning depends upon the child, perhaps even more than the program itself.

I have seen some fantastic progress in oral programs. I have seen some fantastic progress in total programs. I have also seen miserable situations develop under both programs. I have also seen situations, where the programs were very good, but the children were just not rapid learners.

I don't really know if it depends upon the communication system so much, as it depends upon the people driving it.

I sometimes feel we are over concerned with the methods of instruction rather than looking at the child as an individual, and thinking what would be best for him. Lip reading skills, sign language skills, and auditory training skills, should all be evaluated and considered on an individual basis.

This is one of the great weaknesses in our teacher education programs: we do not teach our students how to individualize their instruction. I am not sure we even know how ourselves. But I feel this is an important area into which resources should be channeled.

We also need to realize that it is more important for a child to learn how to read than to attend the state basketball championship. We have to get serious about education. By the way, that is not just a criticism about deaf education, but about our education system as a whole.

Andrew Nielsen:

I think so long as it is not tied into self-concept it is okay. I think this is where the oral schools may have made their greatest error: they tied (lip reading skills) to what the kids should have interpreted as being a key to greater information, to the concept of self-worth.

If one is familiar with how the brain works, the kinetic reinforcement from speech reading is very positive. But it has to be handled in a very de-personalized way. Just because you can't do it, doesn't make you a dummy. Not everyone can be a good speech/lip reader.

Not everyone can be a John Elway. Not all of us can be outstanding quarterbacks. That does not make the rest of us failures. It should not be presented that way either. Our self-concept should not be diminished because we did not achieve the ability of those few who are outstanding.

On the other hand, all of us can learn how to shoot a basketball. We can all learn to pass a football that is fundamentally correct. In this context lip reading training is good. It can take you this far. Then, at some point, natural ability takes over.

I would encourage the exposure to lip reading training as soon as possible. Six months is not too early. It is a part of a total program of auditory training, speech skills, - everything that goes into communication development.

We continue with this in one form or another all the way through high school. We use games and activities to keep it informal. For example, "Tell me what store I am in, from what I am saying." If I say "bananas," it is pretty easy: I'm in a food store. But suppose I say "nuts." That opens a whole list of possible answers: a hardware store, a doctor's office, a psychologist's office, a food store.

But never, never, is the child to get the feeling that if he does not grasp the meaning of these lips babbling, and if he uses sign language to get his message across, that he is a failure. We have done too much of that in the past. We have said signing is a badge of failure.

Helga Simpson:

It is good to be able to lip read to help you survive in the hearing world. But I have read several reports that suggest only a fraction, something like a third of the spoken words are visually understandable, even with training. A lot of the words look the same, and the meaning derived is as much from the context as from anything else.

So, yes, I am in support of lip reading training, but I am also aware that it has a lot of limitations and should be viewed as only a part of a communication package.

Pam Pflueger:

Although it has been stated that only 26% of all words are visible on the lips, I still feel speech reading is very important. Some people are better speech readers than others, but it is important that each child be given the chance to develop her ability as much as possible. Speech reading will depend on the situation. It can be an aid in a noisy environment. It is not a catch-all, but the skill is definitely worth developing so it can be used when needed.

Pauline Zamecki:

It is essential. But be realistic. Don't make it utopian. I can have all the best lip reading training in the world, but if your not talking to me about what I think you are talking to me about, you might as well be talking Greek.

My mother comes into the house and talks to Paula, and thinks Paula understands what she is saying because Paula is a lip reader. This can be dangerous. My mother's lip movements are different from what Paula is used to. Her vocabulary is different. Her approach to a subject is different.

So Paula just stands there and nods her head. It is easier that way and most of the time she can get away with it. My mother assumes that Paula understands because she has been told Paula is a lip reader, when in fact, Paula hasn't the slightest idea of what her grandmother is saying.

Richard Zamecki:

You have to talk in a normal flow of speech. Not too slowly, as that can be as difficult as talking too fast.

Pauline Zamecki:

When I had a gradual and temporary loss of my hearing, I was able to compensate for it by reading my family's lips. I was used to their vocabulary, their sentence structure, the movement of their lips, etc. But when I went outside the family, I was not as successful. My hearing loss was a lot more noticeable. Try turning the television off, and see how easy it is to lip-read the actors!

Richard Zamecki:

I think lip reading training can only help. Sign language does not do you any good in a store. Hardly ever will you find a person who signs and works at a cashier's stand. If you can't find what you want, then you have got to find a way to understand what the person is saying to you when you ask for help. Pencil and paper are always an option, but when it is successful, lip reading is a lot faster.

Ronald Kidder:

I think it is good. We encourage our patients to attend lip reading classes.

Sheila Kidder:

As far as Shannon is concerned, she would probably pass up on the whole thing. Up until four or five years ago she didn't want to talk. She did what she had to do to get by in her speech classes and that was it. Somewhere in the past someone had made fun of her speech, and she decided not to let that happen again.

We were able to overcome that by telling her that, if she would use her speech when she wanted something, then she could have it. I remember one night she wanted a Pepsi. We said, "No, you have to ask for it with your speech." She refused, and didn't get a Pepsi. Well, the next night, she asked for a Pepsi, using speech just as clear as day. Needless to say, we went right out and got her a Pepsi!

This system worked fine until she asked for a horse. We at first didn't understand what she was asking for and said yes. Later we learned that we had committed ourselves to purchasing a horse, and we had to retract that promise! From then on, we were a lot more careful and made sure we understood her speech or asked her to supplement it with signs.

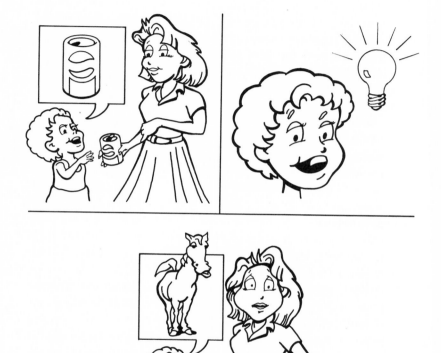

Carolyn Lefever:

I think we should do more of it. Several reports I have seen indicate that this is one area deaf adults wish they were more skilled in.

Are there any special considerations for the home environment with the deaf or hard of hearing child?

Joseph Livingston:

As a matter of safety, I would put in a fire alarm system that uses a flashing light.

I think the security is very important. A lot of deaf children and hard of hearing children that I have worked with have been uncomfortable in the dark. When it gets dark and you can't hear anything you feel even more isolated. I would use night lights in the home.

When I purchase appliances, I would try to get those that showed their functions clearly. For example, I would see if I could get a microwave oven that indicates the end of a cooking cycle by flashing its timer. I would install door bell signals that would flash a light in the house, telephone systems that would activate a light when the phone rings, etc.

I would add carpeting throughout the house. It dampens the echo effect of those noises that are not meaningful. As you amplify sound via a hearing aid, what you need to amplify is meaningful sounds, not the extraneous noises such as feet shuffling and the moving of chairs. Anything you can do to reduce the background noise is going to make wearing of a hearing aid a little more comfortable.

Cheryl Deconde Johnson:

I think the home environment is the place where the child needs to be accepted as he is.

My daughter had a downstairs bedroom. It was quite tiring going up and down the stairs whenever it was time for dinner or when I needed her. So we installed a button in the kitchen that I could push to turn on a lamp in her room to let her know when I needed her. It made life a lot easier for both of us.

Some parents have taken advantage of a Phonic-ear system in which the parents wear a tiny FM transmitter, whose frequency is tuned into a body-style hearing aid that their child wears. Within the limited range of the house, whenever the parent talks, the signal is sent to the child's hearing aid.

I think one of the greatest devices ever invented was the decoder for television.[17] Here a child can be entertained and at the same time see and read English. Word recognition can begin at a very young age. I think the impact of the decoder on reading skills will be phenomenal. I think you will also be seeing benefits to other children who are not necessarily hearing impaired. Those who have learning disabilities and other impairments may also benefit from the visual reinforcement this device provides.

Andrew Nielsen:

To the best of their ability, I think the parents have an obligation to provide those things for the home that make it as rich of an environment as possible for the child.

A decoder for the TV, and a TDD are two things that come immediately to mind. Of course, once that TDD is installed, be prepared for a lot of usage as your child "talks" to all her

---

[17]A television decoder or closed-captioner is an electronic device about the size of a VCR that attaches to a television. It is sometimes referred to as a "TeleCaptioner." It takes advantage of a special broadcast signal that permits it to display, on the lower part of a television screen, the dialogue of what is being said during the broadcast.

Many movies on video tape today are "close-captioned" by placing this special signal on the tape. "CC" on the box indicates this signal is present. Hearing impaired individuals can select these movies to follow the dialogue they would normally miss.

friends! If money permitted, a two line phone system would be the ideal.

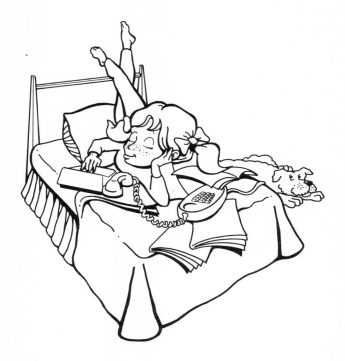

I want to note that other than using signs, we never altered our family's experience because our son, Joel, was hearing impaired. He was a part of our family but the family did not revolve around him.

For many years I would interpret for Joel. For example, at our church services I would interpret the sermons. He probably did more "listening" than any hearing child did. It was only years later that it occurred to me that the deaf person has the right not to watch the interpreter, just like a hearing person has the right to day-dream during a sermon.

Paula Smith:

I would make sure that good lighting is provided. If the deaf or hard of hearing person is attempting to read your lips and can't see them, then it is very difficult to follow the conversation. The same is true for following signs.

The child's room should be his own. He should be allowed to decorate it in a way that is comfortable for him. It is here that he can retreat from the world and relax. Here he does not have to be subjected to the stress of communication. He does not have to read anybody's lips. He does not have to try to follow someone's dialogue. He does not have to worry about signing.

This may be minor but I think for some hard of hearing children a good stereo makes the room more their own. They can listen to their music or feel the vibrations when they want.

I think a captioned TV decoder would be great. It would help tremendously in developing reading skills.

Pauline Zamecki:

Well, we labeled everything in the home: refrigerator, stove, ceiling, window sill, etc. Hearing people know those because they hear it in everyday conversation. Deaf people don't know these things unless you make the effort to teach it to them.

Unless you make the effort to include the deaf child in the family conversations, they will not know about family matters. You have to make the special effort if they are to identify with the family's joys as well as the family's sorrows.

A deaf child is not a real part of the family just because he is born into it. He or she must be actively brought into the family. Sometimes this takes an extraordinary amount of time. I can tell Marsha, my hearing daughter, what I want her to know while I am washing dishes. But I can't do that with Paula. I have to stop what I am doing, get her attention, and patiently explain to her with 100% of my attention what it is I want her to know. Then I have to make sure she understands.

A decoder for the TV is great. Using one, a deaf or hard of hearing child can sit down at the same time as the rest of the family and share a common experience.

Richard Zamecki:

Of course, with the TV decoder, there will be times that your child will want to watch a program that the others have no interest in. Well, that is a part of family life. The deaf child has as much right to watch his choice as the other children. If money permits, get another television.

Your deaf or hard of hearing child is not doing well in school. You suspect that the teacher is not meeting the needs of your child. After going to the school several times and talking with the teacher and supervisor, you still feel the school is not doing a good job. What do you do?

Joseph Livingston:

If my situation is that I have a deaf child in a standard school, then there aren't many alternatives. If his functioning ability is such that his speech is unintelligible, and his language reading ability is low, then we've got some problems. He needs special help. He can not go into a regular classroom and succeed.

I would find another program or move to another community where there was a school for the deaf. Bucking bureaucracy is tough. There aren't too many years of childhood for education; you just don't have the time to try to change a system. If you have tried several times to get the system to address your concerns and have been unsuccessful, then chances are the system is not going to change, at least not in time to benefit your child.

Sometimes the bureaucracy will make it look like you are actually a detriment to your child due to your perceived interference. I would move.

Cheryl Deconde Johnson:

I would sit down and really analyze the situation. If it is a day school mainstream situation with deaf individuals, frequently the interpreter accompanying those students will be the key. That interpreter will set the tone of helping the classroom teacher understand deafness. The classroom teacher will many times shift the responsibility of teaching the deaf individuals to the interpreter. I'm not saying this is right, but frequently this is what happens.

Therefore, I would look at the interpreter - classroom teacher relationship. Do they seem to work together smoothly? Do they support each other? Are they knowledgeable of each other's problems and needs?

When you are dealing with a hard of hearing student who does not have an interpreter in the classroom, then you have a larger problem. As a parent, you are going to have to take the time to visit the classroom more often, to see how you can support the regular classroom teacher. Be aware that when you are visiting a classroom as an observer on a non-daily basis, that you may be very frustrated if you do not understand how the teacher manages his classroom. Try to work with the staff as much as possible.

If the situation is just not working, I would change the child to another teacher. The hearing impaired child can not afford the luxury of wasting a year of education by putting up with a poor teacher.

I would first try to go through the administrative process to get the support to make his change. If that was not satisfactory, I would change schools. You just don't have time to waste.

Unfortunately, I find less than half of the parents of our hearing impaired children really take an active interest in what the school is doing for their child's education. Perhaps a more accurate description would be one-third are consistently supportive in the school and its functions; one-third are supportive on a sometime basis; and one-third leave the education totally to the school.

Andrew Nielsen:
If you are in a mainstream situation, there are always going to be some teachers that are going to say in effect, "If you

can't cut it in this class, you might as well get out." You have to be ready for that kind of response with some teachers. So you find another teacher.

Actually I think that kind of teacher does less damage than the kind of teacher that "smothers" the hard of hearing or deaf student. Some teachers will just shower the pupil with pity and have no expectations for the child's academic performance. That can be very detrimental.

If I, as a parent, can demand that the school educate my hard of hearing or deaf child, then I have the duty to help in that education. It is a shared responsibility.

If it is just a matter of the teacher being lazy, if they are putting money ahead of the eduction of my child, then it is war! Then go to battle!

We have had some battles and we haven't lost yet. We have had to fight individual and group battles, when as parents, we had to deal with situations we felt strongly about.

It helps to have contacts with the school board. Connections help, both on the local and the state level. Reality says you have to go where the power is. You have to cultivate connections. That is how you deal with city hall.

Also, you never gain anything by making another person angry. Threats don't help. If you don't get what you want at the time, make sure you live to fight another day. You can win any battle if you persevere. The question is, "How hard do you want to fight?"

I think many parents become burned-out on the education of their children by the time they are in high school or even middle school. They start out in preschool coming to a lot of the meetings, but after about four or five years of that, they are tired.

Learning and using sign language, constantly trying to improve the home environment, the never ending process of continuing education at home; all of these are very tiring.

This can be especially true when you also have two other children to raise.

Paula Smith:

I would make a lot of classroom observations. What happens in the classroom is the heart of the educational process. Parent-teacher conferences are not enough. Just talking to an administrator is not enough. Parents need to make the effort to see for themselves how learning is taking place inside the classroom. Go into the classroom without advance notice. That will give you a truer picture of what is happening.

If necessary I would start to investigate other schools in the area. I would talk with the teachers, with the support staff, with the administrators. I would question their testing methods. I would see if they had adequate materials. I would observe their teaching methods. Is the teaching time well spent? Again, go in without advance notice to get a truer picture of what is happening.

Then you can make comparisons: how does the school stack up with the other programs in the area? Can things be changed in the school or should you move your child to another one?

Yita Harrison:

I would go and sit in the classroom for several days to observe what is happening. You have got to observe what is going on first hand. Is your child challenged? Is your child at the wrong level? Is he frustrated, and if so, why? How does your child respond to the teacher?

Then I would sit down with the teacher and administration, and discuss my observations to see what could be done. If they are not responsive, I would ask them to respond to the IEP,[18] and if necessary, go to court to have it dealt with. Many parents are unaware of the power they have to fight for the kind of program they want for their children. Because of this lack of awareness, many parents are buffaloed by administrators.

Pam Pflueger:

I have seen this kind of thing happen. The parents are in a delicate situation. I know of one parent who went to the superintendent, but the action seemed to backfire: the teacher resented the parents and other teachers became wary of dealing with the child.

On the other hand, if you feel your child is not being properly taught, you must take whatever actions you feel are necessary. This is especially true with a deaf child because you don't have time to waste. If you can not get your child into another classroom, then find another school. Relocate if you have to.

Parents also need to be aware that changing schools too frequently can be detrimental. My brother was transferred to five different schools during his high school years because the programs were closed due to a funding shortage. The lack of continuity in his instruction made it very difficult for him to progress.

Linda Hawbaker:

When Bobby was three years old he traveled sixty miles each day to and from school, so his days were quite long.

---

[18]IEP stands for Individual Educational Plan. This is a required statement from schools for handicapped children that explains the educational objectives the school has for the child. Parents or advocates review and either accept or reject the proposed plan.

We had some concerns about the teacher before school started and had tried to talk with her. During the year she didn't seem to be able to relate to the preschool kids, and in our opinion wasn't doing a good job. The administration was not responsive to our concerns.

One day Bobby came home with his lunch box still full. I assumed that the teacher must have taken the kids to McDonald's for lunch. It didn't even enter my mind that he could possibly have not eaten all day.

About a week later I asked the teacher about it. She said that he had refused to sit down and do a work sheet, so she did not let him eat lunch. I was shocked. We took Bobby out of the school that day, and he did not return for the rest of the year. It was close to the end of the year, so Bobby didn't miss much school. It seemed to be the only statement we could make at that point.

Larry Hawbaker:

Linda was a lot more aggressive than I was at that early stage in Bobby's education. I was still of the opinion that professionals knew what they were doing. It was only later that I learned that this was not necessarily so. Many parents new to the educational process are at this "they must know what they are doing" stage.

Linda Hawbaker:

I don't think schools knowingly take advantage of that. It is just how the system works. Typically, I will always do everything I can to spend time with a teacher and explain to him my concerns for Bobby. Also, I explain that we will do everything we can at home to support the educational process. This works really well.

But at the same time, we have learned that you have to be willing to take action. If you are not satisfied with the education of your child, then you have to be willing to move your child to a better environment.

Get to know your teachers: Observe, observe, observe.

We tried to move things too rapidly for the system sometimes, and ruffled a few feathers in the process. We did not just sit back and let the system take care of it.

Larry Hawbaker:

We now have Bobby attending both a public hearing school and a deaf school, splitting his days. The attitude of the public school is, "Tell us what you want," whereas the attitude of the deaf school seems to be, "We'll take care of the kid."

Linda Hawbaker:

It's called patronizing. They think we don't know enough to make decisions. They think we don't know enough to make judgments on textbooks. Or what a kid should be learning. Or if they need a curriculum. They don't expect parents to be educated about the needs of a deaf child.

Larry and I went through parent education classes. We were taught in these classes to be advocates for our deaf child. We learned sign language and were taught how to assist in Bobby's education. As a result, our expectations for Bobby's education are high.

Most of our problems were with administrators. They were too removed from the actual instruction of the child. They just didn't know what was happening in the classroom.

As parents we have to live with the consequences of the educational decisions of the school. The administrator doesn't have to deal with this, except during school hours. If a policy is not in the best interest of the child, then who suffers for the rest of his life? The child, and through the child, his parents.

Richard Zamecki:
Go higher up. If you have to, you have to. To get what you need for your child, you sometimes have to fight.

Pauline Zamecki:
You have to dedicate yourself to it. It takes a lot of work. You get tired of it.

Richard Zamecki:
But you do have to do it. For your child's sake, later on in her life, you must fight for her best interests - to prepare her for the time when she will be on her own.

Pauline Zamecki:
Stay keyed-in to your child. There was a stage when Paula was becoming rowdy in the classroom. She was in a school where the teacher so patronized the "poor deaf kids" that she had no discipline. There was no education occurring in the classroom. We knew this had to change, and change quickly.

Richard Zamecki:
Get involved. Meet the teachers. Go and observe what takes place in the classroom.

Pauline Zamecki:

Beware of parent-teacher conferences. They can be a bunch of baloney! A teacher can put up a beautiful front. It is a great opportunity for the teachers to give a big snow job.

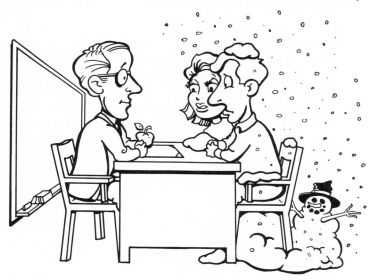

Some teachers will give you the impression that the only problems they have in the classroom is with your child. It is your family that has something wrong with it.

I would strongly recommend that if this is happening with you, that you check other parents and see if they are receiving the same line from this teacher or administrator. Maybe, just maybe, it is not the students who are having a problem as much as it is the teacher.

Sheila Kidder:

Write letters. And make sure that the administrator knows that copies are being mailed to the head of the appropriate departments of education. If necessary, send a copy to your legislative representative, your governor, and others.

Always make sure you have three or four copies going somewhere. Make sure they are going to the people who count. The heads of the various special education departments are a good start for deaf schools, as are budget department personnel.

If need be, you follow this up with appointments and personal appearances. You will get results.

So often, when you get a group of parents together, they will be willing to start by talking with the teacher or an administrator, and maybe even the principal. But that is all they want to do.

You have got to be willing to carry the battle all the way if you are really going to change things. If you are serious about fighting for your child's education, then you have to be willing to go the distance.

Ronald Kidder:

The squeaky wheel gets the oil. If you squeak loud enough and long enough, you will get what you want.

A parent whose child is in the third grade approaches you and asks what reading level can be expected for their deaf or hard of hearing child as an adult. What would you say?

Joseph Livingston:

You have to be careful when answering a question like this. The objective is to help solve problems, not create them. A misleading answer can cause a lot of needless anguish.

I would be honest. If you work really hard at it, your child can be a good reader. If you don't work hard at it, then your child will probably end up reading at a third grade level as an adult.

If a lot of parents really believe in the value of reading, then teachers will believe in reading. It is just like sports: if the parents in an area believe football is important, then usually there is a good football program. You just can't wish it into being. It has to be supported with time and commitment. It is up to the parents.

Reading and language are a lot different than math. Math achievement levels are usually higher, extending up to the seventh or eighth grade levels. Math is a more concrete medium that is pretty straightforward.

Math concepts are not as difficult as language syntax, structure, and meaning. True, initially language is simple. For example, the word "table." "A table," "this is a table," "on the table," "under the table," "above the table," are phrases that are easily understood.

But when you move up to concepts like honesty, then you are getting into the abstract, which is more complicated. Reading for content, reading for inferences, and reading for meaning require a lot of understanding over and above simple word definition.

Cheryl Deconde Johnson:

I think a lot of that depends upon the parents' involvement with their child at home. The expectations for reading achievement run anywhere from third or fourth grade to high school.

Given that you have normal intelligence, it will depend upon how much communication you have at home that supplements school. Language and English both affect reading. If you have a good language base, then you are going to read a lot better.

I do think the telecaptioners will dramatically improve reading levels. The Signed English systems are going to help also, but the biggest single factor will be parental involvement and the priority that reading achievement has in the home.

Andrew Nielsen:

I would say to the parent, "How much time are you willing to spend on it?" If you are willing to give them outside experiences as a basis for reading, then the sky is the limit. They could read right along with their hearing counterparts.

It is the parents that make the difference. The school does not have the resources or time to give them the language base for reading achievement. The parents need to do that, along with the brothers and sisters.

Donald Kitson:

I think a fifth grade reading level would be a reasonable expectation. Most parents are shocked when they hear that. Unfortunately they are not informed of this fact until their child is within a couple of years of graduating from high school.

It is a shame because most parents wish they had known this years ago, and if there was anything they could do about it. The school should tell the parents early enough to prepare them for this possibility.

In an imaginary graduating class of fifty seniors, it has been my experience that maybe ten will go on to college. Of those, only one third will actually finish four years of college. That is three students out of fifty.

Frequently, this is because the schools do not really train their students how to study. The schools are not strict enough. The tests are too easy. The students pass to the next grade level with very little real effort. I must add though, that I can not place the entire blame on the schools. The parents, too, must take an active interest, and expect their child to develop good study habits and self-discipline if they want their child to succeed. The school can not do it all alone.

The use of television decoders helps improve the language level, but this should be used only after school, and after the pattern of finishing homework first has been established.

Without the parental support the child has little hope of being prepared for college.

Yita Harrison:

As a language and reading teacher, I have had that question posed to me frequently. It is hard and dangerous to predict the future.

I have had instances where I felt there was no way a student was going to make it to college. Then while the child was still in high school, he suddenly blossomed, and became a very good student and did go on and succeed in college.

I have had other instances where I believed a student was college bound, only to later see him waste away on drugs. Or he became tired of school and quit studying. Or, or, or, ...

So I have become very cautious in making predictions. Predictions can turn around on you.

I do advise parents that there will most likely be a three to five year reading lag between their deaf child and his hearing contemporaries. This is due to the difficulties encountered in language development.

For example, my own hearing children were speaking basic sentences in correct syntax when they were one and a half years of age. Many of our deaf children start school at three years of age, and are just learning single word definitions. They are already two to three years behind their hearing peers in language development. A very, very small percentage of these deaf children will ever make up this difference.

Pam Pflueger:

I wouldn't want to limit a child. His reading level will depend largely on parental involvement and ultimately on his own motivation. I would impress on parents that without their active instruction, it will be difficult for a deaf child to improve his reading level.

Linda Hawbaker:

I would say to the parents, "You are the ones who can make the difference. Whether you get involved will probably be the deciding factor."

Larry Hawbaker:

The school just cannot do it all. Sure, you can be very lucky and have a really good language and reading teacher, but still that is only for a limited time during the day. A fourth grade reading level is the norm more often than not.

Linda Hawbaker:
The education is both a school and a home function. A really good teacher only gives you, the parent, a brief vacation from teaching the child yourself.

I would venture to say that most of the informal, unwritten curriculum in elementary education occurs at home. The school provides the guidelines, but you as a parent must take an active teaching role with your child if you really want that child to progress.

Larry Hawbaker:
Hearing schools seem to be more strict. If you don't know the math tables by fifth grade, then you can very possibly remain in fifth grade for another year. In deaf schools, the attitude seems to me a lot more lax: "Well, maybe he will get it next year."

Linda Hawbaker:
Normal deaf students should be held accountable before progressing to the next grade level.

Returning to your question, I would say without any special help from the parents, a fourth grade reading level is an appropriate average expectation. With parental involvement, this is not a limit. Right now, Bobby's reading level is past high school. This took a lot of extra effort on our part. A lot of people in our family worked with Bobby.

Richard Zamecki:
Try to tell the parents that the reading level will only be as good as the effort they put into it. With a deaf or hard of hearing child, you have to put more into it. You have to really help them with reading.

Pauline Zamecki:

You have to be realistic about it also. Your reading level will correspond with your speech or signed vocabulary. If you have learned good sentence structure in English, then you will read well. If you are a deaf person who has a limited speech or signed vocabulary and sentence structure, then you really can't understand what you are reading.

I can not comprehend some things that I read because the people who write them are so sophisticated, that they can not write at my level of understanding. Their vocabulary level and sentence structure is such that I just don't understand what they are trying to say. That makes me a poor reader in their environment.

If a deaf person is reading at the third grade level, then he is going to be a poor reader in the high school environment.

I have read several studies that argue that reading is a verbal, not a visual task. If that is true, then the deaf have a big strike against them: they do not have the verbal skills, they do not sign in exact English, they don't even communicate among themselves in exact English. So how can they read English easily and understand what was written?

If your deaf child can read the newspaper, at least he or she is functionally literate. I believe that is around a fifth grade reading level. This reading level is achievable if the parents are willing to make the extra effort. Paula reads the newspaper all the time.

I do feel that goals are not set high enough in schools for the deaf. Too often the attitude is, "Well, they are deaf, they can't read well, so let's not try to teach them anymore than we have to."

Richard Zamecki:

It all comes down the old saying, "the more you put into it, the more you are going to get out of it."

Pauline Zamecki:

Reading takes practice. You have to keep doing it. With the effort there is no limit. You, as a parent, have to be a teacher also.

I remember keeping a journal for Paula. Everyday I would write the activities that Paula did during the day. I would write a short story and try to draw pictures of what we did.

For example, "Paula ate two eggs and toast for breakfast." I would write that sentence, and then draw a picture of Paula doing just that. Then I would go over that with Paula.

I would send her home journal with her to school. Her teacher would then reinforce the language with Paula in school.

Her teacher would also create a school journal of her class activities. She would write what they did in school that day, and we would go over that with Paula when she got home. It was a constant, daily team reinforcement.

Richard Zamecki:

Another indicator would be to go to the school and find some high school students who have the same level of hearing loss as your son or daughter. See what reading levels they are functioning at. Then get to know the parents and find out what they are doing, and how much they are working with their children.

Pauline Zamecki:

You also have to be realistic. Each child is different. Some will achieve more than others. But if you want your child to have the chance to read above the third grade level, you have to commit the time and the effort as a parent. It won't just happen.

Richard Zamecki:

As I look back, there was a lot of extra effort, but it sure was worth it. People who meet Paula now can't believe she is profoundly deaf. I am very proud of her and her accomplishments.

Sheila Kidder:

If you are lucky your child will be able to read at the sixth grade level.

Had I known that when Shannon was in an earlier grade, I would have gotten some outside help and worked a lot more with her.

Shannon is a very intelligent girl. She has passed her SAT tests to be accepted into college, but she is at the very bottom level. She will be the last one accepted. Something is wrong with the standards if this happens, and she is getting all A's in her classes.

For example, Shannon is taking chemistry and getting A's. So we told the college that she applied to that she had an A in chemistry. Later we found that she was only on page 42 of her text after three months of the school! How well do you think she is prepared for college? This is educational fraud or something very close to it.

Parents have got to demand high standards for their children. You can not wait until your child is a junior in high school to realize this. You have to fight for it back in the elementary school and all the way through.

Carolyn Lefever:

The statistics say that on the average deaf kids graduate with a fourth to fifth grade reading level. I would say to the parents that they are doing the right thing, thinking about this, investigating it now, and not waiting until their child is in high school.

If they want their child to be truly literate they will have a tough row to hoe. Their child must be able to speak or sign English in order to read it well. Otherwise the child will only be picking up words here and there; hopefully putting two and two together; and guessing correctly about the meaning of what she has just read.

Their task will to be to insure that a lot of communication is happening at home, preferably in English. If not in exact English, at least moving towards exact English. This emphasis will have to continue for years and years without let up.

I would recommend reading "experience stories"[19] at home and reading with the parents in fun situations. I recommend tutoring during the summer months.

Finally, as a teacher, I would keep in contact with the parents and encourage them to keep going. Don't give up. You will make the difference in the reading achievement level of your child.

---

[19]"Experience stories" are stories written by a parent or teacher, that tell of the child's activities during the day. They are then used as a tool for language instruction that the child can relate to in a personal way.

A parent approaches you in panic. His child is graduating next year and still can't read at the fifth grade level. What would you say?

Joseph Livingston:

There is always hope for the future. If the parent, and more important, if the child wants to take additional steps to continue a reading program, then great.

There are numerous programs that offer reading programs for adults. These might be successful if there is a strong desire on the part of the student. I would encourage the parents to go to the programs and see what they offer. I really don't know from first hand experience.

The largest problem they are going to have to deal with is the motivation of their child. If the child is not motivated, then I doubt whether any of this would do any good.

There are many factors that go into the process of learning to read. I am afraid we don't understand that process very much. For that matter, we don't understand the process that goes into hearing very well, let alone reading. We seem to have basic ideas, and feelings as to how you learn to read, but we don't really understand why a person doesn't learn to read.

If suddenly at seventeen or eighteen, the student wants to learn to read (or greatly improve his reading), I think it can be done.

Also, quite frankly, I would think to myself, why the sudden interest in the child's reading ability? Where were you three or four years ago? Certainly by seventh or eighth grade your child should have been reading.

I feel reading is the primary task of our educational system. Without reading, a person doesn't have much chance in today's world. I think reading is the area where we should put our bucks in the educational process, particularly in educating the deaf.

I might add, I have not seen a good program, in my years in teaching the deaf, that deals with the employment picture.

We talk about it. I've seen some canned programs out there. But I have not seen a sequential program, starting out in the kindergarten level, that helps a deaf child figure out what he wants to do in life.

Cheryl Deconde Johnson:

I would hope this would not really be a surprise to the parents. I would like to think that the parents have been active participants in their child's education over the years; that the parents have been attending parent/teacher conferences and know pretty much where their child stands.

What we need to do, then, is sit down and look at the child's achievement levels realistically and see what is best from here. What are our options? Do we enter the child in a junior college and have him take some classes in remedial reading? Do we say the child has reached his reading level potential? Do we need to look at vocational areas where reading is not emphasized?

Andrew Nielsen:

I would say, "I think we (the school) have done a pretty good job with your child. At least 50 percent of his peers are reading at a level below fifth grade, so he is not doing too badly. True, approximately forty-nine percent are reading better, but what did you as a parent do, during the last ten years?"

If you will remember, when you came to me when your child was in preschool, I advised you that if you didn't make an intensive sign and communication effort with your child at home, he was not going to progress beyond a fifth grade reading level. So if he is in fact at that level now, I know you didn't make any great efforts at home to go beyond this, and I would suggest that you get off my back.

I do feel the telecaptioners will be a tremendous boost for deaf kids in their reading skills. I think in four to five years, deaf kids will knock the socks off the reading scores of today.

Getting back to the original train of thought, I think that by the time a student is fourteen, he pretty much understands whether he is reading well or not. At some point, it becomes the student's responsibility to understand that the more you do something, the better you get. If he really wants to learn, he is going to have to make an active effort.

Though there are post-secondary courses available for the adult who wants to learn reading, at this point it will be up to the student whether this is a priority or not.

Paula Smith:
I would like to respond to that question in terms of a vocational evaluator. The colleges for the deaf today are allowing students to enter with a seventh grade reading and seventh grade math level. Sometimes with intensive tutoring, the students can elevate their SAT scores to this seventh grade level. This would probably take about two years, and would take a tremendous amount of study and tutoring.

I would recommend the child have a complete vocational evaluation. That would consist of mechanical tests (for fingertip dexterity and gross motor movement analysis to determine technical program feasibility), office and clerical tests, and interests tests. This would give the parents a more objective picture of what their child can and can not do.

If the child reads at the fifth grade level, chances are he would have a very tough time in the college environment. Technical programs such as carpentry, electronics, or food service would probably be a better way to go.

Yita Harrison:

Though illiteracy is a product of deafness, a person's reading level can always be improved.

I have a friend who has a thirst for knowledge. She graduated from a residential school back in the 1950's. She has always felt she has never had enough education. While she was raising a family, she never had time to improve herself. She asked me, "How can I improve my vocabulary?" I encouraged her to do crossword puzzles and read.

I would take her to the library and we would select books, starting with fifth grade level materials. Every three months we would return to the library and select another group of books that were a bit more difficult.

To satisfy my curiosity, I gave her an SAT test before she started her work. She tested at the 5.8 grade reading level.

Two years later, she had improved to a 9.9 grade reading level. Now she loves to read.

Another woman comes to my mind. She was in my adult education reading classes. She tested at a grade 1.3 reading level. She was in my class because she couldn't read the directions the doctor had written out for her, on how to take care of her sick baby. After three years, she left with a 5.0 reading level. She was twenty years old and she wanted to learn.

I feel there can be improvement no matter what the student's age, but the person has to be motivated.

Pam Pflueger:

Hopefully the parents have been involved with their child's education, and this should not be a surprise. I would stress the kinds of vocations that their child could pursue with his particular abilities, and the training programs that are offered.

If the child was motivated and the parents were interested, I would suggest appropriate local contacts for remedial courses. The Model Secondary School (MSSD) at the Gallaudet University Campus has a program called P.E.P., Post Enrichment Program. It is an intensified program in English, reading, and math for those students who have not made the necessary entrance exam scores to be accepted into college, but have shown potential and have demonstrated a desire to further their academic education. But it is important to enroll in this program immediately after high school graduation, because the child must be twenty-one or under when he begins the program.

A lot of what happens depends on the motivation of the child. One high school teacher discouraged my brother from taking an automotive mechanics class because of his reading level. He was so determined to get into this class, that he studied on his own and later proved to the teacher that he could indeed learn the necessary technical jargon. He got into the class and excelled.

Larry Hawbaker:

I would hope this would not be news to the parents. I hope that someone would have told them when their child was small, that most deaf children achieve only a fourth grade reading level by the time they graduate.

I still remember being told about reading level expectations and it was a shock to me. Bobby was two years old at the time. I feel we were very lucky that someone told us: if we wanted Bobby to read at a level higher than fourth grade, we were the ones who would have to work to make it possible. I believe Bobby would be no higher than the fourth grade level if we had done nothing.

Linda Hawbaker:

I don't have a whole lot of sympathy with a parent that has not been aware of this possibility for many years. I'd ask them where they had been during their child's education.

Carolyn Lefever:

I'd be tempted to say, "Where have you been the last ten years? You are a mite late with your concern." I know this is just a venting of my feelings and might be counterproductive, but it is what I would like to say.

Since the student is graduating, he is probably close to being an adult. If the student and parents have a good relationship, the parents may be able to influence the student to participate in tutoring. However, if the student and parents have a poor relationship, I'm afraid the parents have missed their chance.

A parent approaches you in panic. Her child is graduating next year and still can't do fifth grade math. What would you say to her?

Andrew Nielsen:

Math is different than reading. Find out where the student has trouble: was it in understanding content (labeling such as "pounds," "ounces"), in computation, or in application? These are the three main areas to be concerned with.

We are finding out that most hearing impaired kids do pretty well in the content area, and very well in computation. It is in application where they run into problems.

Application involves more abstract processing. For example, you go to a store and you need to buy a large quantity of beans. The sign says, "Two eight-ounce cans of beans for $.30." But you also see a sixteen-ounce can for $.32 . Which is your best buy?

The kids can probably read the signs. The problem is in processing the information, developing and executing a plan.

As the symbolic representation for a meaning becomes more and more abstract, it becomes more difficult for the person who has a limited understanding of our language and its structure to process language-based problems. If the natural language of the deaf is a concept/pictorial language, there will be difficulty when abstraction takes place. A morpheme - based language, on the other hand, would simplify the understanding of these and other related comprehension tasks. This would be especially true in many math word problems that demand precise understanding of the meaning of each word in a sentence. Algebra, geometry and higher math courses are loaded with these abstract concepts.

Yita Harrison:

I strongly believe the school tried its best. Maybe the child was not motivated to learn. Education is a two way street between the school and the child. It takes efforts on both parts.

Linda Hawbaker:

I would not be as concerned about math as I would about the reading. With calculators kids can do the math without mastering mental computations.

Of the two, reading is a more powerful tool. It opens the door to education, jobs and money. If there is a lag, reading would be my first concern.

Pauline Zamecki:

Your child is normal. Math scares a lot of people. If he understands what math is all about, the child will not stay at the fifth grade level but will move on. At this stage, he probably just doesn't understand math concepts.

Richard Zamecki:

If a child doesn't know how to do math with a calculator or a computer, then he's got some real problems.

Pauline Zamecki:

The problem isn't that people can't add five and five and get ten. The problem is in processing the information in a work situation. If I need three pieces of something 45 inches long and a yard and a half wide, how much do I need? That is a real problem for a lot of kids. It is not adding two and two. It is knowing that you need to add two and two in order to solve the problem. Kids need to know how to use numbers to get to where they want to go.

Sheila Kidder:

Get a tutor, a good one. A correspondence course won't work for more advanced math because you need someone to guide you and answer your questions.

Get into the school and find out why your child has not learned more. Question the school. If people don't get into their school and make demands on the school, then their children are probably not going to get a good education from the school. I don't care if it is a regular public school or school for the deaf. If you have a problem, go to the school. If you don't go, it will never change.

Carolyn Lefever:

My response would be the same as to the previous question regarding reading: if the student is willing to accept tutoring, fine. If the student is not motivated to accept tutoring, then the boat has left the harbor.

What vocations would you suggest for the hard of hearing or deaf student who has just graduated from high school. He is definitely college material, and has absolutely no idea of what he wants to do in life?

Joseph Livingston:

There are several questions that must be answered by all students: Do they really want to go to college? Did they go to school every day because they liked high school or because they had to? If they didn't like high school, then they should question whether they will be successful in college. Remember, college is school.

Secondly, do they know what they want to study? I think the best way to find out is to go out and try jobs in different areas. Try to experience the field before committing yourself to the time and expense of years of study. There is nothing like working at a job to give you a feel for exactly what goes on in that field.

Actually the answer to that question really is no different for a deaf child than it is for a hearing child.

Cheryl Deconde Johnson:

This is career exploration, and it varies from student to student. It is wide open. Of course, you should suggest fields to avoid in which deafness would pose an obvious hardship.

The National Technical Institute for the Deaf (N.T.I.D.) in Rochester, New York, has a wonderful program for deaf college students. I did an internship there and was greatly impressed. They prepare students for the working world by teaching them practical skills.

The students are allowed to explore various practical fields, rather than a general liberal arts program. Too many times, I feel the general liberal arts program is a luxury that does not really prepare the deaf individual for working.

My own daughter wants to be involved in space exploration. She wanted to be an astronaut, but because of her hearing loss she could not qualify for an astronaut training program. She understands that.

However, she may be able to do other jobs to get into space. It is possible that she could be an engineer on a flight. Although she would not be in the capacity of an astronaut, she would still be involved in the program.

She has done waitressing. This summer she is a cashier at an amusement park. So she is doing things that make her use her communication skills. She occasionally has problems, but she is learning how to cope with situations that demand good communication skills.

Her major in college is astronomy. She is now studying in Tucson, Arizona. She is struggling. The math is difficult and she has gotten a tutor to help her write her papers.

She will be a sophomore this fall. Whether she will be able to make it or not, I don't know, but she sure is trying. It is what she wants at this time in her life.

Andrew Nielsen:

What is so sacred about college? How about a better word, "vocation."

Baking is becoming a lost profession.

Forensic specialists could easily be deaf. Imagine a trained visually orientated person arriving on a scene of a crime. The visual skills and knowledge of what to look for would be perfect for deaf people.

I really don't like the idea that the deaf must go into computers. There are a lot of other very satisfying occupations that the deaf can be involved with.

My son, Joel, has changed his job ideas several times. First he wanted to be involved in sociology, then he wanted to be a biology teacher, and now he wants to explore landscape engineering. I feel he would be great in psychology. There are so many different things he could do well. He is like a kid in a candy shop: he just can't make up his mind. How many people really know what they want when they are eighteen?

I have heard that fifty to sixty percent of the jobs that will be opening in five years do not even exist now. So what difference does it make what I say now?

I feel that if we got together and decided to become good Danish bakers, in three years we would all be millionaires! There is so much virgin territory out there waiting for a good Danish baker.

Don't be afraid to use your imagination. Don't think in isolated channels. Think of what is best for you.

I remember I spent eighteen years of my professional life trying to get my dad to accept my vocation. He always equated success with salary level. Using his criteria, as a teacher, I am not much of a success.

Just before he died he was at our home when we had a party for a group of deaf students. He sat though that party and when it was over, he said through tears in his eyes that he understood what I was doing. After eighteen years of seeking his approval, he finally understood the kind of work I did. That meant more to me than making a million dollars.

So, I guess a person has to sort out what is important to him in life. If it is making money, that is fine. It is okay to make lots of money if that is truly what you want. Each person has his own idea of what will make him happy. No one else can make that kind of decision for you.

Paula Smith:

He should have some idea by the time he graduates as to what he would like to do. Hopefully, in his educational program he would have been exposed to various job ideas. His educational, vocational, business, and sports classes should

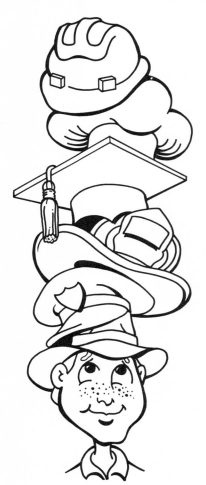

have given him a taste of each of these areas.

He could take interest tests. He could also look through job dictionaries. These books describe various jobs, their salaries, their educational requirements, and the working conditions.

Work experience during the summer months is very important. Even volunteer work broadens the student's idea of what goes on in different jobs. It also gives the student a good opportunity to develop good working habits, interpersonal skills, good grooming habits, and so on.

Working after school during the school year helps. Anything that adds to the child's knowledge of what goes on in the working world, will help him decide what he wants to do later on in life.

Realize that students will also change their minds from year to year. Vocational evaluations are good to help students get into the habit of evaluating what they want to do; and what they would have to do to get into a field.

These evaluations also help a student make a realistic choice given his abilities and educational background. If the parents want more opportunities for their child, they will have to work on that from the beginning. The senior year in high school is too late to find out how low the reading or math level of their child is. Parents should watch their child's progress throughout his education.

Yita Harrison:

I think most deaf people are initially quite happy with their jobs. Unfortunately I don't believe they get the advancement they deserve as time goes on. The main reason, the old excuse goes, is because they cannot use the telephone. Another, is that the deaf person does not have the communication skills to supervise hearing people. This eliminates the possibility of the deaf person gaining the experience of being a foreman, or rising into management. This is something to consider when choosing a field: what are the advancement possibilities, given my handicap?

Larry Hawbaker:

I would suggest to a student that he try a junior college. Explore different classes. It is cheaper and usually not as difficult as going to a university.

Linda Hawbaker:

We have never had any preconceived ideas of what we wanted Bobby to do. We did want him to have the background skills, to be able to study and do whatever he wanted.

I really don't think it is appropriate for a parent or a teacher to pick a vocation for the child. That is up to the child to decide.

I am glad Bobby has experienced a mainstream situation in high school. He is attending the high school math classes at the local hearing high school. There he is able to get the look and feel of competing with other hearing students. I feel this can only help him be better prepared for college.

When Bobby entered his early teenage years we allowed him to explore ideas. As a part of the normal growing process during this time, we encouraged him to think independently. So we feel that as he continues to grow, he mentally and emotionally will be better able to make decisions like selecting a vocation on his own.

Helga Simpson:

I would say expose the child to as many different job training situations as possible. Through experiences during the school years, it is hoped the child will get some idea of the types of vocations that he would want.

I would never have any recommendations for any particular vocations for the deaf. That is up to the individual. I would not want to steer him with my biases. I feel most fields are open to a deaf person if he sets his mind on it.

Pam Pflueger:

I would not want to limit a person. I know of two hard of hearing individuals, who are in successful sales positions that involve constant communication with the public.

Two areas that are multifaceted, are the graphic communications field and computer science. Through my experiences in job development, I have found these fields to be of interest to hearing impaired people because they are able to utilize their visual learning skills.

I feel that vocational programs for deaf students reading at the third to fifth grade level, really need to be expanded to include additional remedial classes. These programs also need closer coordination with private industry.

The National Technical Institute for the Deaf (N.T.I.D.) at the Rochester Institute of Technology (R.I.T.) in Rochester, New York, provides an excellent technical training program for hearing impaired students.

The Program for Hearing Impaired (P.H.I.) at Northern Illinois University in DeKalb, Illinois also has a good vocational exploration/training program. The Northern Illinois program instructors are all certified teachers of the hearing impaired. This can be a great benefit for those students who are in need of additional remedial help beyond the scope of an interpreter. Contact your vocational rehabilitation office and request assistance from the counselor for the deaf. Be aggressive!

Patty Pittroff Swain:

I would recommend a good business education. That is what the whole U.S. commercial world is all about. With a general business background, you can later branch out into anything you want. But follow your heart.

Richard Zamecki:

I would think a lot of the deaf population would be able to successfully get a job working at a bank, working on 10-

key machines and things like that. Really any job where the communication level is not a high priority would be appropriate.

Construction is not that good. It can be done, but it is difficult. There are a lot of hazards that could be very dangerous if you couldn't hear.

Also, you would have to be able to receive and understand a lot of instructions from your supervisor: get the wrong figures and there could be some real problems.

Sheila Kidder:

I am a firm believer that deaf people can do anything they want to do. That includes becoming lawyers, doctors, or anything else they want. They may require an interpreter, but if they want to pursue something badly enough, then it is possible.

Carolyn Lefever:

Well, I always wanted to be a cowboy or a vet, and there was a stage where I wanted to be a porpoise trainer! It is such an individual thing, I really can't say what vocations would be best.

How do you feel about hearing individuals marrying deaf individuals?

Joseph Livingston:

The ones that I have known have had a tough time. The reason is communication. It is a big problem.

I have had a deaf individual tell me he would never marry a hearing person. When I asked why, the response was that he couldn't tell what the hearing person was saying on the telephone. Many deaf individuals feel they can't trust a hearing person, when they can not monitor what is being said.

It is the same feeling hearing people have when they see a group of deaf people signing at a table. They don't understand what is being said and become uncomfortable with the situation.

Cheryl Deconde Johnson:

I don't have any personal experience other than seeing some of my former students who are deaf, marry hearing people. I think it is a very individualized thing.

The hearing person has to understand that he will be asked to do a lot of translating and communicating for his spouse. He has to be willing to make this extra effort and understand the incredible responsibility this implies.

My daughter has only dated hearing boys. My daughter can speak, but she does know and use sign language. She is currently dating a hearing boy. He is learning sign language because they find they can communicate easier with it.

Kids are unpredictable. Five months ago she said she would never get married and wanted to live alone on a space station. I have learned with kids, what they say one day can completely change on another. They are predictable in their unpredictability.

I must add that when she used to go to the Aspen Camp for the Deaf, there were two weeks in the summer where she was surrounded with people like herself in their deafness. For two weeks she did not have to meet the expectations of the hearing world. She would always come back so relaxed. I think this experience is a critical one to remember: when she was with others who were deaf or hard of hearing, she was surrounded with a comfortable social and emotional support group.

Would I go so far as to say she should then marry a hard of hearing person? I don't know, that is up to her. If the person has the right qualities and is hard of hearing, then I think it would be easier for her than marrying a hearing person. But, again, the decision will be hers.

Andrew Nielsen:

I would rather see my deaf son have an inter-racial marriage to another deaf person than to marry a hearing person. There are just too many obstacles.

I do not want Joel to be a plastic model that performs at hearing parties. "Oh, how wonderfully he functions!" I don't want his hearing wife to be dragged to deaf social functions where she may feel totally out of place. I have only seen one deaf/hearing marriage work half way.

Paula Smith:

Well, I am very hard of hearing and my husband, Chuck, hears normally. We have been married over two years and we get along just fine.

I think it depends mostly upon the communication skills of the deaf person. If the person has good communication skills then there is a reasonable chance that the marriage will work. At the same time the hearing person has to be aware and accept the limitations of deafness. For example, when you are driving in a car and the interior lights are out, it is very difficult for the deaf person to communicate. The hearing person will have to realize that the deaf person will want to socialize with some deaf friends. He will have to accept that.

I think a deaf person who depends completely upon sign language will have a tougher time. Signing requires more of an effort. Will the hearing person always be willing to make this extra effort?

When we rent movies, we try to find movies that are captioned. My husband has learned some signs, but since I function well orally, we rarely use sign language between ourselves. I do not really need to use signs to understand my husband. We are lucky in that communication between us is not a problem.

Chuck Smith:

I know that when I talk to Paula, I have to face her. I have to make sure the light is good so she can see. There are times I have forgotten to do these things, but we both seem to be able to correct problems with a sense of humor.

I want to learn more signs. I am especially aware of this need when Paula has her deaf friends over. There are times I can not understand what is going on at all.

Paula Smith:

It is also difficult at times for me to keep up with the hearing company that my husband has, but that did not prevent me from marrying him. It all depends upon the individual. The qualities of the individual and the compatible interests are more important.

Chuck Smith:

I do not view the fact that Paula is hard of hearing as being a threat to the marriage. As a matter of fact, half the time I forget that she is hard of hearing. She is so good at lip reading it is amazing.

Paula Smith:

I know I function more as a hard of hearing person, even though I am very deaf. Many people ask me as to whether I am hard of hearing or deaf. Ninety percent of the input I get from a person is from reading his lips.

Our marriage is a happy one, but again, I function more as a hard of hearing person.

Donald Kitson:

I feel that in the short run a marriage might work, but in the long run it would not. At first the flame of love is hot, but over time it burns out. Social situations are different. Families are different. These are two different worlds.

I do not believe I could successfully marry a hearing person. A deaf woman would better understand my needs.

In the movie "The Children of a Lesser God" it was interesting to note that the hearing teacher of the deaf children did have patience with the deaf children. But would he be able or willing to extend that patience, to a twenty-four hour basis with a deaf wife? That is a very good question to ask any potential hearing spouse of a deaf person.

Linda Storch:

If a hearing boys's parents are deaf and he marries a deaf girl, then that would be okay. He would know what deafness was like because he grew up with it. He would know what he was getting involved with.

I have seen situations where a hearing girl marries a deaf boy to become his "mother," to take care of him. It seems to start out fine, but in the long run it just doesn't work. In the end her patience runs out.

I remember one time I had a hearing boyfriend. I would feel sorry for him when he had to stand while I was signing to my deaf friends. I really didn't like that. And when I tried to follow what his hearing friends were saying to me, I was frequently frustrated and lost. It was no fun.

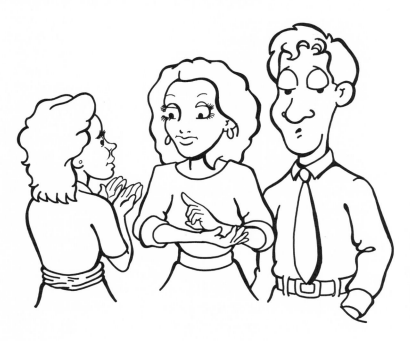

Yita Harrison:

I have seen a lot of that. I would say maybe 2% are successful. And in these 2%, the hearing partner was raised in a deaf family - either the mother or father were deaf. They grew up in the deaf culture and they feel comfortable in the deaf world.

Other than under these circumstances, I have never seen a deaf/hearing marriage work. This is due to communication problems.

First there is love, romance, and sex. Later on the interests are different. The deaf person wants to associate with his deaf friends for communication and friendship. The hearing person wants to be with other hearing people for the same reasons.

The hearing person will want to listen to music, go to movies that are not captioned, and go to plays. The deaf person has no interest in these, and over time it takes a toll on the relationship.

I have seen the hearing children in such marriages virtually ignore the deaf parent. It is easier for the children to communicate with the hearing parent. This leads to jealousy, fighting, and divorce.

Linda Hawbaker:

Well, I think it would work, but it really depends upon the two individuals. Sometimes I feel the deaf attract hearing people with a certain kind of mentality. The "poor little deaf child," the patronizing kind of attitude is not what I want Bobby to have. Many hearing people look at the handicap and not at the individual. Some hearing people can be so caught up in sign language, and want to be a part of it, that they loose sight of the people they are dealing with.

Larry Hawbaker:

I have seen it so many times: the hearing population sees a TV program that sensationalizes the young deaf boy who says, "Mom," for the first time, and all of a sudden these people want to save the deaf and become teachers of the deaf.

Linda Hawbaker:

Many times to the hearing world this deafness is new and different, something to be played with and explored.

This is especially true for many religious groups. I feel the deaf are especially susceptible to joining such groups because they are not normally welcomed by the hearing world. But then here comes an organization that pays a lot of attention to you.

I am sure most of these organizations mean well, but there are times when I feel this little undercurrent of "what we are doing for the deaf." I feel the deaf are better left alone to do for themselves.

Getting back to your original question, the hearing person would have to be pretty aware and patient. I have seen it work, but the deaf person has to have his own profession so he is not too dependent upon his hearing spouse.

Helga Simpson:

I see how comfortable my daughter is with other deaf individuals. I would prefer that she marry a deaf man because I feel she would be more comfortable.

I feel it would be very difficult for a hearing person to have the patience required to be married to a deaf person. Imagine the hearing husband coming home from the job tired. The deaf wife has been home all day and is just dying to rap and talk with him. Signing requires a lot of effort. He is tired and just doesn't want to sign. He wants to relax. There could be some real problems with that.

Pam Pflueger:

It depends upon the individuals involved. I do believe it is possible to have a successful marriage, but it would be difficult. It can be very fatiguing for a hearing person to repeat things over and over. Using sign language and a TDD require a commitment of time and patience for both parties. It is difficult for the hearing person to always be an interpreter.

Some deaf friends have told me that signing can be very tiring between two deaf people, and even more exhausting when signing with a hearing person. A deaf person would have to be very patient with a hearing partner whose natural language is not sign language.

I knew one hearing impaired person whom I considered having a relationship with. He had excellent speech reading skills and a fantastic command of English. In spite of this, there were times when the energy level required to continue a successful dialogue was exhausting. Because our personalities differed a lot, we had difficult moments. These were compounded by communication barriers.

Patty Pittroff Swain:

Well, I am in my second marriage. My first marriage was with a deaf man. My second marriage is to a hearing man.

Every individual is different. Though I am hard of hearing and know sign language, you would think that my first marriage should have worked out. Unfortunately, my first husband had too many personal problems that overwhelmed the marriage. The deafness was not a factor.

It is hard to say. It is a very personal thing. You must have a very understanding mate. If my second marriage should fail, I would not rule out falling in love with another deaf man or with a hearing man. If the love is strong enough, I could marry anyone.

As I think about it a little more, I realize it would require a lot of patience from the hearing person to make it work. Sign language is a real effort.

Richard Zamecki:

I think a deaf/hearing marriage would be helpful for the deaf person, if the hearing person has the patience.

Pauline Zamecki:

I think it is a cultural question. Can a black person and a white person have a marriage and survive?

The deaf person has his world, and the hearing person has her world. Can they combine the two?

I think any two people can make it in a long haul situation if that is what they make up their minds to do. But it will require a lot of give and take. It will require the hearing person and the deaf person to accept each other as people. Accept what made you that kind of person and what will continue to mold you as a person.

It would be very hard to break the communication barrier. I think the patience required by both partners would be almost overwhelming. It could be done but those two people would really have to dedicate themselves to each other.

Richard Zamecki:

I think if the deaf partner was really plain, then maybe the chances would be better because the hearing individual would be truly interested of his partner. It wouldn't be a matter of good looks, as over time that would be not enough to support the marriage.

Sheila Kidder:

Well, ninety percent of the time I am totally against it. Too many times it is tokenism.

I have seen it so often. A hearing boy likes Shannon and decides to learn sign language. He enjoys showing her off to his hearing friends. He is dating this cute deaf girl. Sooner or later the novelty wears off and the boy returns to his hearing world.

The hearing person has so many things to understand. Not only to learn sign language, but to learn the deaf culture and deaf psychology. The amount of understanding required is just immense.

If you are not deaf yourself, then learning about the deaf is like learning about another country. It is not only the language of this country that is different, it is the entire culture that is different. Does the hearing person really understand this?

I know when I am really tired, I can't even understand sign. When I get this way, I tell Shannon that, and she either writes things down for me or signs very slowly. Will a deaf person understand this when a hearing spouse feels the same tiredness? Will the patience be there over the years?

Ronald Kidder:

Another question: will the deaf and hearing partners grow intellectually at the same rate over the years? I feel on a daily basis, the hearing person absorbs a lot more than the deaf person. It is just because the hearing person receives so much more input because he can hear. This is a potential problem for the marriage in the long term.

Carolyn Lefever:

I think it would be a pretty tough situation, especially the feelings of isolation when among the spouse's friends.

How would you summarize the differences between the hearing world, the hard of hearing world, and the deaf world?

Joseph Livingston:

That is a hard question. These are only my general impressions.

The deaf world is much smaller than the hearing world and it has a tendency to be cliquish. The privacy among the deaf sometimes seems to be relatively limited. It is like a small town with almost no secrets.

I feel the hearing person is never fully accepted into the deaf world. The deaf feel the hearing never really understand, and they are probably right.

I have seen many instances where the hard of hearing person who can cope with the hearing world, is permitted to lead the deaf group during those times that they need his services, but after this need is fulfilled the hard of hearing person is returned to a fringe status.

I am not an advocate of deaf power. I feel it has a tendency to isolate, and one thing the deaf do not need is more isolation.

The hard of hearing world requires a lot of adjustments. Those who seem to have the hardest time are individuals on the fringe of the deaf world. They might be close but still have too much hearing to be accepted into the deaf world. Try as they might, they are never really accepted by the deaf world.

I think the hard of hearing individuals who elect to try to be a part of the hearing world are much happier. Many times it is frustrating for them but as a whole I feel they are happier.

Andrew Nielsen:

The hearing world and the deaf world are distinct, and in that sense they are the same. My heart really goes out to the hard of hearing individual. There is really not a hard of hearing world. The hard of hearing person spends most of his life trying to find identity in one of the other two worlds.

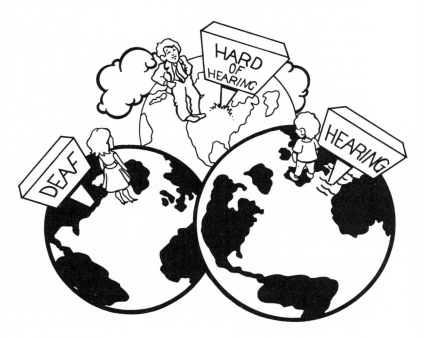

Paula Smith:

In the hearing world you have maximum opportunities to communicate.

In the hard of hearing world you have some opportunities to communicate, some opportunities for socialization, and some opportunities for educational achievement.

In the deaf world you are talking about an entirely different culture. They have their own language. They definitely depend upon a different mode of communication, either total communication or sign language.

I know of some deaf individuals who have tried to be in the hearing world. Usually these are individuals who do not want to admit that they are hearing impaired. Frequently they are very frustrated individuals.

I think there are many interpreters, who through their knowledge of signs try very hard to be in the deaf world. They, too, are frequently frustrated because the deaf world does not accept them.

For the most part the deaf world also refuses to accept hard of hearing individuals. I think this is because the deaf world resents the fact that hard of hearing individuals have greater opportunities open to them. To the deaf, even outward appearances seem to suggest that the hard of hearing person is more successful.

I feel that the typical deaf person has a better self-concept than the hard of hearing person. The deaf person belongs to a group and he knows his limitations. The hard of hearing person faces a lot of isolation. He doesn't belong in either the deaf world or the hearing world.

Donald Kitson:

The hearing and the deaf worlds are as different as black and white. The hard of hearing world is like multiple shades of grey.

The divorce rate is high among deaf individuals. Their choice of spouses is relatively limited. This leads to many mistakes.

Patty Pittroff Swain:

They are each separate worlds.

The deaf world is very cliquish. If you don't fit into it, they let you know right away.

The hard of hearing person has it especially hard. He doesn't fit into either world. The hearing people will not want to repeat a sentence, and the deaf will not want to repeat a sign.

Larry Hawbaker:

I think there will always be a social barrier between these groups. Even if the deaf person can read well and be as knowledgeable as his hearing contemporaries, he will never really socialize with them.

Linda Hawbaker:

I do feel these barriers are being broken down somewhat through the use of computers and modems. Bobby is very capable in using the computer and through a modem he is able to "talk" with other people.

For instance, Bobby can call a person in Ohio and "talk" with that person, and that person has no idea that Bobby is deaf. The person Bobby is communicating with might be a quadriplegic - and Bobby has no idea about that either!

Pauline Zamecki:

I think the deaf tend to be more paranoid. They are always sure someone is talking about them. They feel that someone is always trying to make a fool of them or take advantage of them. Even among their own deaf friends this seems to be a problem.

They feel they are always under observation by the hearing world and that the hearing world is always criticizing them. Though this is frequently not the case, the deaf perceive it that way.

Sheila Kidder:

Deaf adults in the deaf community are very often very suspicious of the hearing. Often they feel that they have been taken advantage of by hearing people.

Hard of hearing people are not as suspicious as they are intimidated. Everything that is said they take personally. If they hear it, they perceive it in a negative way directed towards them. If they don't hear it, then they are convinced the conversation was about them.

Many times hearing people look upon the hard of hearing people and deaf people as being stupid or ignorant. They don't understand the difference between not being able to hear and not being able to learn.

Carolyn Lefever:

I think of the hearing world and the deaf world as two distinct societies. The hearing world is the larger society with the most opportunities. The deaf world is the smaller of the two groups with fewer opportunities. It also is a tighter social group. I see the hard of hearing world as a fringe group of both these two worlds.

Any closing thoughts to parents and teachers that you would like to add?

Cheryl Deconde Johnson:

I think hearing individuals are guilty of saying what they feel is best for the deaf and for the hard of hearing, without really knowing and understanding what these two worlds are all about. We have got to listen more to these groups and to learn more about the feelings of these two groups.

I would have done a lot of things differently as a parent, knowing what I know now. I would have taught my child sign language. I would have had made it a point to have established good communication at the earliest age possible.

My daughter and I really didn't communicate well until she was six years of age. This is too late. If she would have had language input at an earlier age, I think the first five years of her life would have been much easier.

It is very important that our hard of hearing and deaf children are not isolated. This has a great deal of bearing on their self-esteem.

First, accept your child as a child. Sure there is the handicap of deafness, but always deal with the child as a person.

Give your child every benefit you can. Consider moving to a good program if one is not available in your community. Get the hearing aids and other devices for the home that would improve his language input.

Have a strong commitment and participation to the school that your child is in. Show the child, by your example, that you believe that a good education is important for his future.

The child's communication skills will largely determine how far he will go. Though not every deaf child will develop good oral communication skills, most of them can develop a basic ability to express their needs.

Provide as supportive an environment as you can. Spend as much quality time as you can educating your child.

Incidental learning is not going to happen. You need to be redundant. You need to teach things over and over. You have to be consistent.

Too many times I disciplined Jenny out of frustration before we had learned sign language. When you discipline your child, make sure you can communicate with the child so the discipline has meaning.

Andrew Nielsen:

Language is so very abstract. It is so difficult to accurately describe a steak that is cooking on a charcoal grill. You can try thick, juicy, smoked - but you really have to experience it to sense what it is.

It is only after experiencing something that the words describe that language assumes some approximation of meaning. Language growth is tenuous at best without these experiences and the coupling of the experiences with the appropriate words.

The deaf have the experiences but the language meanings are not introduced at the same time. The hearing child passively picks up word meaning and language by hearing them when things happen. The deaf child must be actively taught to associate a sign and a word with an experience.

The social cost of this handicap is enormous. I think this is especially true for the hard of hearing individuals. They constantly have a problem of trying to feel comfortable with either the deaf world or the hearing world.

Author: I have posed the question to several of my deaf students, "If you had to make the choice, would you prefer to be deaf or blind?" Many responded that they would rather be deaf, because at least they could see colors.

Andy: Yes, but is it worth the isolation?

Author: Speaking for myself, yes, because I do not feel I can depend socially on anybody. As a result of my experiences of being hard of hearing, I don't trust completely: I don't "trust" that I can follow the dialogue of a conversation, and I have extended that to my social relationships.

I know I can see colors and those colors don't emotionally hurt. If I was to trade that ability for being able to hear completely, I would be at the mercy of people hurting me.

Because I am hard of hearing, I have viewed all my social interactions as being either (1) challenges to understanding dialogues, (2) threats of being made a fool of, or (3) tremendous and exhausting efforts required to keep up with a social situation. Frequently, it is easier to be alone.

I would rather have my vision because I would not need to depend on people. If I wanted to socialize with someone I could do it with sign language, at least with other deaf people. If someone hurt me while I was socializing, then I could withdraw and I would still have my sight.

Andy: If I had to be born either way, I think I would prefer to be born blind. I want to be able to talk to people. I basically trust people. I know all of us have "feet of clay," we all have shortcomings.

I know that when I open myself up to people I am opening myself up to hurt; but I am also opening myself up to joy. I am opening myself up to anger; but I am also opening myself up to agreement. I think sometimes many people with a hearing loss don't understand that we all have the same feelings. Everybody is human.

In the past I have put many people on pedestals. I really looked up to them. Then they would do something very human. For a long time I was really angry with them for not being what I thought they were. It was only over time that I have realized that all people are only human. It was my mistake to try to make and expect them to be more than what they are. People are people and their mistakes will involve hurt.

I think at this stage in my life, given the choice, I would rather lose my hearing. I would want to retain the ability to see. Because I have my language, I can communicate with people. If I were born blind and never saw the sunset, it wouldn't make any difference to me. I would still be able to acquire language and communicate with people.

The deaf are more isolated than the blind. You see a lot more marriages between a hearing person and a blind person, than a hearing person and a deaf person. The successful union of two people requires a good communication base. One of the worst forms of punishments is solitary confinement. To be denied social contact with your fellow human beings is terrible.

As a parent, I have never viewed raising a deaf child as being a burden. As I reflect upon my life, I think it is probably the most enriching experience I could have had. I have learned more from my deaf son than I have ever taught him.

I am not going to say there were not times when I wished I did not have to sign. There were those times when I was talking with my wife, and Joel would walk into the room. I would start signing.

I had feelings of wishing I didn't have to sign, but I'm not going to feel guilty about feeling this way. I am a human being, and I am entitled to being tired of signing.

Frequently after I would start signing, the beauty of his intellect would come out as he joined in the conversations. This was very satisfying.

Handicap is an attitude. We expected Joel to do everything his siblings did. He was never able to play for any special sympathy from us, so he never learned to use his deafness as an excuse.

Deaf power is an expression of immature militancy. There you see an attitude of "treat me differently" that I just don't agree with. Deafness, the handicap, is given more emphasis than the individual. That is not right. It conveys a feeling of a negative uniqueness. I hope all my children feel unique, but I don't agree with a negative uniqueness.

Yita Harrison:

I think hearing people should note that the deaf are sometimes quite limited in their language. So when they say something it comes out quite direct. The deaf do not have the subtle vocabulary the hearing use to make a point. This is unfortunately interpreted as being without tact but really is only due to a limited language vocabulary.

Helga Simpson:

Treat your child as a normal child. Do anything and everything you would normally do with a hearing child. This includes discipline. That is the best advice I could give any parent of a deaf child: don't treat the child differently.

Also, communicate with your child whenever you can. Use sign language. Have a happy, positive, loving attitude, and your child will pick up on that and return it to you. Have patience with yourself as well as with your child.

Pam Pflueger:

Deafness affects your ability to communicate. A deaf child will have difficulty learning the intricacies of the English language. Even deaf adults with a good command of English language find that everyday situations can be frustrating: seeing a doctor or a loan officer, buying a car or a house, getting directions, ordering food in a restaurant.

There will be ample opportunities for frustration and pain on everybody's part. When I chose a birthday card for my brother, I used to wonder if he would be able to understand the subtleness of the joke inside. In turn, when he chose a Father's Day card, did he understand the message that he was giving?

It is not easy to deal with deafness. Including a deaf family member in activities and constantly explaining things is very tiring for the entire family. My father had a particularly difficult time. When my mother passed away, the responsibility of raising my brother fell largely on his shoulders. He wanted to provide support for his child, but the inability to communicate often overwhelmed him and he frequently felt defeated.

Some families I know would sometimes hang up on an incoming TDD call when they knew their deaf family member was not at home, because they were intimidated by the TDD machine.[20]

I have seen families become frustrated during television programs when they were asked by a deaf member to explain what the dialogue was about. This frequently resulted in arguments because the deaf person wanted to understand the program, and the hearing family members did not want to be interrupted and have to interpret the program. They felt there was no escape from the demands imposed by deafness, even in watching television.[21]

---

[20]For those with the financial means, a separate phone line and number for TDD calls could be installed in the home. In this way, then the phone light(s) went on, it would obviously be a call requiring the use of the TDD.

Today's latest TDD's come equipped with message recording capabilities. With this and a separate line, the child would not have to rely upon the parents or family in regards to the phone even for messages.

[21]Television captioning decoders will greatly help alleviate this problem. The text of the television conversation is displayed on the screen. There will probably be times when the deaf child will want the parent to explain some sentences the child does understand. As the child's language level increases, this should decrease.

Sports can be very beneficial in developing a bond between a father and deaf son and enhancing self esteem. However be aware that deafness can lead to withdrawal from participating in sports with hearing kids. My father had to really encourage my brother to overcome this. Some deaf children will require a lot of extra encouragement to overcome their fear of not being accepted because of their deafness.

If the standards set for the child either by himself or by his parents are too high and the child repeatedly falls short, he will eventually give up trying. You can't fail if you don't try.

Parents are the key to their child's success. Consistent academic, emotional and social support from both parents will determine your child's development.

Learn as much as you can about your child's needs. Learn about the psychology of deafness and how hearing impairment can affect your child's self-esteem. Insecurity, lack of trust, and isolation are very real among some deaf people.

If you have a young deaf child, participate in parent-infant training programs.[22] Go to workshops at a school for the deaf. Get to know your local centers for the hearing impaired; the hospitals that have speech pathology and audiology departments; the schools for the hearing impaired; and the local universities that have speech and language departments. Contact the John Tracy Clinic in Los Angeles. They have a mail correspondence program for home study. Contact Tripod, a preschool for the hearing impaired whose philosophy is a Montessori approach. Contact the Alexander Graham Bell Association for the Deaf, the American Society for Deaf Children, the Convention of the American Instruc-

---

[22]Some national organizations that provide literature and advice on parent-infant training programs are The American Society for Deaf Children, The Alexander Graham Bell Association for the Deaf, the National Association for the Deaf, and the National Information Center for the Deaf at Gallaudet University in Washington, D.C.

tors for the Deaf, the National Association of the Deaf, and the National Information Center on Deafness.[23] If there is nothing available locally, then I would greatly encourage a move to a location that can offer support.

Don't hold your child back just because he is deaf, that is false protection. Allow your child to experience failure, but be there to guide him through these failures as learning experiences. Your child will need constant and consistent positive reassurance that you believe in his abilities. Self-doubt can be paralyzing. Sometimes this encouragement may seem harsh. But as in disciplining a child, a spanking can sometimes be of more benefit than ignoring the problem.

I remember my parents would sometimes reward my brother if he finished his homework by taking him to the local Dairy Queen for an ice cream cone, but he had to order the ice cream cone himself. Many times he refused to do this. He was scared to speak. There were many nights he would go home without a cone if he refused to try to speak, while the rest of the family had one. At the time I thought my parents were being very cruel. At some point he decided that the cone was worth the effort and overcame his fear of speaking to get a cone.

Years later we happened to be driving by that same Dairy Queen. He spotted it and asked me if I remembered it. Then he told me he'd buy me a cone. He not only ordered the cones but made a date with the waitress!

Get your child involved in activities in which both of you actively participate: bowling leagues (child/parent teams), dances, community projects. Associations of the hearing impaired have a wealth of social activities that you can become involved with. Include activities that are fun, to build up a reservoir of good times you and your child have

---

[23]See appendix for a complete listing of names, addresses, and telephone numbers.

shared. Obviously, positive reinforcement on your part is a key ingredient in this.

Involve your entire family. When you are teaching your deaf child, teach your other children how a deaf child learns. It is important to make the other children aware of their deaf sibling's needs and to make the other children realize they are important in assisting in this educational process. When my brother was young, my mother gave us the option of attending his preschool and working with his teacher. We did so daily during the summer months for three years, and we enjoyed learning how to participate in teaching my brother.

Install all the assisting devices possible in your home such as a TV caption decoder, flashing alert signals for the telephone doorbell or fire alarm, and TDD for phone use. If nothing is available locally, contact Harc Mercantile, Ltd. They have over 450 products for the deaf. Sunburst Communications has recently produced captioned videos on topics that are very important during the teenage years such as education on drugs, nutrition, and building self-confidence.[24]

Understand that as your child reaches adulthood, your ideal of a date for your child will not necessarily be what your child wants. The population of the deaf community in any given locale is usually so small, that the opportunities for meeting deaf dates is quite limited. Initially my father preferred that my brother date girls of the same religious background. Later he realized how difficult this was for my brother.

The deaf world, the hard of hearing world, and the hearing world are each different. Each have their own perspectives. No individual in one world has the experiences of what it is like to live and cope in the other worlds. Therefore, we must be cautious in asserting our personal agenda when we try to cross from one world into another.

---

[24]See appendix for a complete listing of names, addresses, and telephone numbers.

Patty Pittroff Swain:

Growing up, the hard of hearing child will not feel that he belongs many times. Parents should watch out for this, and try to help the child feel he can be a part of a group. This applies to the preschool child as well as the high school student.

Many times I remember watching the children in our neighborhood playing games. I would have very mixed emotions. Sometimes I would want desperately to go out and play with them. But there were other times, I would rather not, as I knew that I would be laughed at and talked about because I could not hear everything. It was quite lonely at times.

I was in an oral program, but wish I had been in a total communication environment as I was growing. I feel I lost a lot during my high school years. I always liked men teachers better because it was easier to understand their deeper voices.

During my high school years it was frequently just easier to withdraw because it was so hard to communicate. I became very shy.

Linda Hawbaker:

I guess the biggest thing I had to learn was to trust myself, my feelings, and my intuitions about things.

I had to get over the feeling that just because someone is a professional she knows what is best. She may know a lot and know different things than you do as a parent, but she does not always know what is best for your child.

Surround yourself with a support group of other parents and teachers who will share their concerns and feelings with you. Frequently you will find common concerns and can help each other in searching for ways to solve them.

Very often parents believe something is not right, but they feel they are unable to do anything about it. They frequently are so insecure about their own intuitions that they do not back up their beliefs with any meaningful action.

If you believe in something strongly enough, especially when it involves the education of your child, you will succeed if you put forth the effort. Find parents who have children the same age as your child. They will have concerns for their child similar to your concerns for your child.

I would encourage parents who have children in the lower schools to contact parents whose children are in high school, and ask their advice for ways to prepare their child for the coming years. Prepare yourself as much as you can about what you can expect and how you can improve your child's education.

Speech development was never one of our priorities. Bobby is profoundly deaf. When Bobby was very young, we visited other profoundly deaf teenagers and we saw what to expect as far as speech went with this group.

Associate directly with deaf high school students. This will expose you to their concerns and frustrations. In this way you can try to head off similar problems in your family.

For instance, I remember seeing several high school students who were left out of their family's dinner conversations. I decided I would not let that happen while Bobby was growing up, so we learned sign language.

Other times, I remember seeing deaf children who were not able to watch TV with the other members of the family. As soon as the television decoders came out, we got one for Bobby so he could read and enjoy the same programs we watched. The circle of language and reading is so important; one reinforces the other.

It is tough to educate a deaf child. A young deaf child is like an empty chalk board - you must consciously put language and experiences into the child. He does not absorb words, speech, and language in a passive way as a hearing child does. It all must be actively taught to the child: names, events, dates, everything.

School is not enough. You have to continue reinforcing education at all hours of the day. You, as parents, must become teachers. Also you, as a parent, will know more about your child than any school administrator or teacher. It is just common sense because you spend more time with your child than anybody else.

Parenting is so very tiring with a deaf child. It is physically and emotionally exhausting. Signing requires a lot of patience and effort. Constantly teaching and explaining things to your child is exhausting.

It can break a marriage, but it can also bring a marriage much closer together. Working for a common goal can make your lives so much more interesting and enriching. Of course, this assumes that both people really accept the deafness and agree to tackle the problem in the best interest of the child.

Everybody marvels at how bright Bobby is. Bobby is a normal child. He has just received a lot more input than many other deaf children. We made it a point to teach him at home and follow his progress during his school years. Deaf children can be more successful if they receive greater input from their parents when they are young.

Sheila Kidder:

We don't even like the word handicap. We prefer to call it a challenge.

Your child can do as much as any other child. Let your child know it. If you treat them differently than your other children, they are going to think they are different. Then you have handed them a crutch, an excuse, for thinking they can not accomplish something.

We have always told Shannon she is not handicapped. She can do anything anybody else can do. You may have to do it differently, but you can do it - just find your way.

As far as discipline goes, each child, hearing or deaf, is different. We use a dialogue/discussion approach with all of our children. We always give the reason we are taking some action or making some decision. We then give each of our children time alone to think things out. Each of our children handle this differently.

Shannon will frequently come back within a half an hour and say she is sorry, and that she accepts the decision that was made. One of our other children will take two or three days to finally accept a decision and stop pouting.

Recognize that each child is different. The hearing or deafness is only a part of the whole child. You have to deal with the whole child.

Perhaps because we always had five or six children around, there was never enough time to treat Shannon differently. If she touched something she wasn't supposed to, she got her hand slapped just like her brothers and sisters. Of course, each of the siblings think the others receive too much attention, but that is just normal sibling rivalry.

Shannon would occasionally test us but we were aware of what she was doing. Any child is going to test you regardless as to whether she is handicapped.

After we had Shannon we definitely wanted another child. We did not want her to be both the deaf child, and the baby of the family. We felt that position had too much potential to cripple her. We wanted the new baby to divert our attention so that Shannon would not be the center of attention. We wanted her to learn to share.

Open up and give your child love. These children are not different than any other children. If you give them love, you will get it back many times over.

CHAPTER III:
FORMER HEARING IMPAIRED STUDENTS

INTRODUCTION TO CHAPTER III

Too many times the published views of what the deaf want, or need, or feel, do not come from the deaf population, but from a professional that works with the deaf who is actually voicing his own opinions. While it is not my intention to suggest that professional views are to be dismissed, I believe there is a need to listen to what the deaf themselves have to say about how they were raised and educated.

The interviewees in this group are quite young, between sixteen and twenty-four years old. The memories of their childhood and the interactions with their parents, siblings, teachers, and other students are still quite fresh in their minds. Time has not had a chance to diminish their praise for jobs well done, nor has it had a chance to soften their sometimes harsh criticism.

Though all of these young adults are hearing impaired, the hearing loss is about all they have in common. Each participant is unique, not only in the hearing loss itself, but also in personality, mental and physical abilities, and family background.

Some of these young adults are hard of hearing, others are profoundly deaf. Some have very good speech, others have very limited speech. Some are very skilled lip readers, others rely exclusively on the use of signs.

Each of their families have dealt with the hearing loss in a different manner. Are any two families the same? Some parents accepted the loss and aggressively moved on to minimize its effects. Some parents never accepted the loss and even today do not accept the whole child. Some parents learned sign language, some did not. Some insisted that their children go to oral-based schools that did not allow their students to sign, while others sent their children to schools that permitted and even encouraged the use of signs.

All of these young adults have attended special schools for the deaf at some point in their education. Some were in these schools only very briefly. Others have attended these special schools throughout their education.

At times some of the responses to the individual questions seem to diverge into other areas. Nevertheless, I felt it was important to preserve the emphasis, and the content of the participants' responses. For this reason the answers were generally kept intact as they were recorded. The author has taken the liberty of editing the responses to present them in a more easily understandable form.

At times the answers to a question seem to be repetitious. At the risk of being redundant, I included these responses to show the common thread among the participants.

There are other times when opinions varied considerably. This is natural whenever a group of individuals is surveyed.

This group and this section does not pretend to speak for the deaf, but it does add an important dimension to this book.

I wish to thank these young people. They willingly contributed their time and their thoughts, so that others might benefit from their experiences.

THE PARTICIPANTS

John Saddler
Profoundly deaf
Loss occurred at the age of five due to spinal meningitis
Both parents have normal hearing.
All siblings have normal hearing.
Twenty-four years old
Currently attending college in Phoenix, majoring in mathematics.

Tami Saddler
Hard of hearing, cause unknown. Progressive in nature, possibly hereditary. Loss could become profound in the near future.
Hearing loss was first suspected when Tami was eleven. It was not fully recognized until Tami was sixteen years of age. At that time she entered a special school for the deaf.
Both parents have normal hearing.
Other siblings have normal hearing.
Twenty-two years old
Currently employed as an auditor for Circle K Corporation.

Tina Priest
Severely hard of hearing since birth due to mother's rubella during pregnancy. Loss is stable and has not deteriorated further since birth.
Both parents have normal hearing.
All siblings have normal hearing.
Twenty-four years old
Currently a homemaker with an eighteen-month-old son who has normal hearing.

Lulu Sinsabaugh
Profoundly deaf
Born with normal hearing.
Hearing loss occurred at eight months of age due to spinal meningitis.
Both parents have normal hearing.
Has three hard of hearing sisters, one is Roxanne Ruiz, another participant.
One sister with normal hearing
Twenty-three years old
Currently married to a deaf man. They have a three-year-old son who has normal hearing.

Roxanne Ruiz
Hard of hearing, 55 db loss in left ear, 60 db loss in right ear
Loss occurred at age of three due to illness.
Both parents have normal hearing.
Has three sisters who are hearing impaired: Lulu, a profoundly deaf older sister who is also a participant, and two younger sisters who are hard of hearing.
One sister with normal hearing
Seventeen years old
High school student at the Phoenix Day School for the Deaf

Paula Schurz
Severely hard of hearing: right ear (65 db loss), left ear profoundly deaf since birth, due to mother's rubella during pregnancy.
Hearing loss was diagnosed when Paula was two years old.
Both parents have normal hearing.
All siblings have normal hearing.

Twenty-three years old
Currently works part-time for a publishing company. Paula is married to a severely hard of hearing man. They have a two-year-old boy who has normal hearing.

Shannon Kidder

Profoundly deaf since birth
Both parents have normal hearing.
All siblings have normal hearing.
Twenty years old
A college freshman at the National Technical Institute for the Deaf in Rochester, N.Y., majoring in photographic arts.
Shannon recently competed in several track events at the Deaf Olympic Games in Australia.

Debbie Pruett

Profoundly deaf since birth due to mother's rubella during pregnancy.
Both parents have normal hearing.
All siblings have normal hearing.
Twenty-three years old
Currently working full time as a library clerk at the Central Library in Phoenix, Arizona.

Kathy Ferguson

Severely hard of hearing since birth due to mother's rubella during pregnancy.
Both parents have normal hearing.
All siblings have normal hearing.
Twenty-two years old
Currently attending N.T.I.D., majoring in accounting.

Lori Little
Profoundly deaf
Loss occurred at eighteen months of age due to spinal meningitis.
Both parents have normal hearing.
All siblings have normal hearing.
Twenty-two years old
Currently attending Mesa Community College in Mesa, Arizona, in a general studies program emphasizing business and computers.

Jennifer Simpson
Profoundly deaf since birth, cause unknown.
Both parents have normal hearing.
All siblings have normal hearing.
Twenty-three years old.
Currently attending college at N.T.I.D., majoring in applied accounting.

THE INTERVIEWS

Imagine you had to inform parents that their child was deaf. What would you say to them?

Tami Saddler:

Although the child has lost his hearing, he should be able to live a normal life. Though the loss of hearing is a factor that now must be considered in raising the child, it should not be considered as an overwhelming limitation.

The child's brain works just fine. He is not mentally handicapped and is certainly not helpless. You will be able to communicate with your child. His language can be developed either orally through lip reading or through the use of signs. Many deaf and hard of hearing people use a combination of both methods.

The child could attend a regular public school, with or without the assistance of an interpreter. If the services are not sufficient, there are schools for the deaf that will assist you in his education.

I personally would recommend the use of signs. It helps in vocabulary development. I would also encourage the parents to develop the child's oral skill so he will be better prepared for the hearing world.

Roxanne Ruiz:

I would be scared for the parents. It would be so new to them. They might have a lot of fears and imagine a lot of things because they have had no experience in dealing with deafness. I would try to reassure them that deafness is not the end of the world, it just means that their child can't hear.

I would tell them, though, that if they really want to communicate with their child they should learn sign language. I would encourage them to contact other parents who have deaf children for their advice and support. I would also tell them to get in touch with a school that deals with the education of the deaf. I would give them some phone numbers of several other people who know about deafness who could help them by answering their questions.

Shannon Kidder:

I would encourage the parents to go to a school that would show them how to teach their child speech and signs. This is commonly called total communication. It involves using all the means available to establish communication between two people. This includes using signs, speech, lipreading, and gestures.

I think it is important for both parents to learn sign language and to teach this to their child as soon as possible. If both parents learn sign language, then both parents will be able to talk with the child as he grows up. Communication between the parents and the child will have an early start.

Debbie Pruett:

If I knew what caused the deafness, I would try to explain to the parents how their child became deaf. I think it would be easier for them to accept the deafness if they understood what caused it.

Kathy Ferguson:

If the child has any hearing left at all, I would encourage the parents to get a hearing aid on the child as soon as possible.

I would tell them not to be afraid of the deafness or of their child. She will be more normal than they might think.

I am severely hard of hearing and I am successful in school. I play sports, I work, and I enjoy the same things that hearing people enjoy.

Lori Little:

I would tell the parents that their child is deaf and not to panic. The child will be able to do a lot more than they realize. Deafness can be dealt with successfully.

Jennifer Simpson:

Except for the fact that their child is deaf, the child will be normal. He will grow up and experience the same problems, joys, and frustrations as all children.

Do you remember any misunderstandings that occurred when you were very young which you later realized were the result of your hearing loss?

Tami Saddler:

Many times I would say words wrong or say them backwards. I remember calling my uncle "Feeheart." Later, I realized that I was supposed to call him "Sweetheart." Nobody corrected me on this because they thought it was just baby talk.

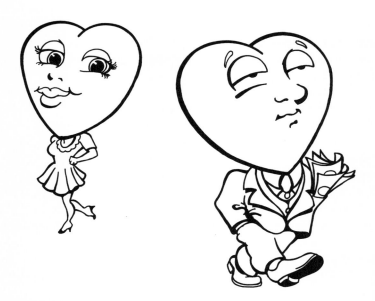

Tina Priest:

I remember running out into the street as a little girl. All the people in the cars were honking their horns, but I couldn't hear the horns or what the people were saying to me. I didn't understand what was wrong. Luckily my mom heard the horns and came out and got me before there was an accident.

I remember another time when our family dog bit my brother in the face. I think it was because my brother had been teasing the dog. I remember trying to tell the dog that he had been a "bad dog." When I think back on the incident, I wonder what the dog thought of my efforts. I had no real speech at that time.

Lulu Sinsabaugh:

When I first went to school, I watched people making odd movements with their hands. I didn't understand why they were moving like that. It was only later that I realized this was a way to express meanings, to communicate ideas.

Roxanne Ruiz:

I remember being put into the corner by a teacher. She was very frustrated with me because I would not do what she said. She thought I was just being stubborn. She didn't know that I couldn't hear her when she called my name, or that I couldn't understand what she wanted me to do.

At the time I thought everybody had the same problem. I thought everybody could hear - or not hear - as I did. It was only later that my parents learned that I had a hearing loss and placed me in a school for the deaf.

Paula Schurz:

When I was young I was enrolled in a program for the hearing impaired. The teachers would stand very close to me. I didn't understand why they were so close to me. I wanted to tell them to back off a little. It was only much later that I understood they wanted me to watch the movement of their lips and repeat their speech patterns.

Debbie Pruett:

When I was very young, I used to watch people talk. I didn't know what they were doing. Why stand and move your lips? Later, I understood it was a means of communication. I wanted to say "Mother" and "Father" with my lips, but I didn't know how.

I remember when I was about three or four I didn't understand the word "dead." When the word was used I just laughed. I thought it was funny to see people sleeping that way. What a silly waste of time! Nobody had explained the meaning of the word "dead" to me. It was only later that I realized that death was not the same as sleeping.

Kathy Ferguson:

When I was young and people said things to me, I didn't understand. I felt I didn't know anything at all.

It was only later that I realized I was not dumb. I just didn't hear the message clearly, and that is why I didn't understand.

Lori Little:

I remember going to my father and trying to sign to him. I thought everybody was the same, and that if you signed to them, then they would sign back to you. Well, my father didn't understand my signs. I felt like such a fool. Later it dawned on me that hearing people do not normally use signs to communicate.

I also couldn't figure out why they didn't understand me when I spoke to them. If they could talk to each other, then why couldn't they understand me when I talked to them? Why were they making things so difficult? Was I the brunt of some game they were playing?

It was only later that I realized my speech was different. Among other things, being deaf meant that my speech was not clear.

Jenny Simpson:

I remember I always had to point to things to get them from my mother, things like milk or cookies. I noticed my brother did not have to point. He would just move his lips and my mother would get him what he wanted. This puzzled me.

It was only later that I realized I could not tell my mother what I needed or wanted. We used our own system of signs to communicate between each other. Later these signs were supplanted by conventional signs.

How old were you when you realized you were deaf?

John Saddler:
I grew up deaf, so I never thought of myself as being deaf or different. I am who I am, and that is normal for me. I can not remember thinking, "Oh, I am deaf and different from the hearing world."

Tami Saddler:
It wasn't until I was fifteen that I really had to accept that I was losing my hearing. At that time people started telling me that I could become completely deaf. I didn't know anybody who was deaf. I was scared.

Tina Priest:
One day when I was about five years old, I came home from the deaf school I was attending. I was learning sign language at the school. I noticed my brother was talking to my mother and not using sign language. I asked my mother why he didn't use sign language like I did. My mom responded, "...because your brother is not deaf." I realized then that there was something different about me.

Roxanne Ruiz:
It really hit me when I went to the deaf school in first grade. I saw a lot of hand movements that I had never seen before. And the noise level in the classroom seemed a lot lower than it had been in kindergarten. I realized then that my hearing was below normal. But my older sister was completely deaf and going to the same deaf school so I wasn't very upset.

Paula Schurz:

When I was in fourth grade, I finally understood why the teachers would bring their faces so close to mine and say, "Watch my lips!"

Shannon Kidder:

When I was about three years old, I noticed people talking and I couldn't hear them.

I also remember encountering the word "deaf." I asked my mom what it meant. She said it meant that I couldn't hear any sounds. At first I didn't understand what that meant.

A little later I watched my family communicate by moving their lips. They understood each other. I understood nothing. After a short while I put the two together and realized I didn't understand, because I couldn't hear the dialogue.

Jenny Simpson:

I remember watching my brother move his lips and letting my mother know what he wanted, without using gestures or sign language. Why couldn't she understand me when I said something? Why did I always have to point to something I wanted?

Later I realized that my mom didn't understand me because I couldn't talk very well. I didn't know how to pronounce words. I couldn't understand what the lip movements meant. No matter how hard I tried, I could not attach meaning to the motion. That was when I realized I was deaf. I guess I was about five years old.

What frustrates you most about being deaf?

John Saddler:

In a word, classification. The hearing world classifies people too much. Black. White. Polish. Deaf. Blind.

The hearing world rejects us in a lot of ways. One example is jobs. Another is social activities.

I believe the hearing world perceives the deaf as being incapable. They see only the handicap. They do not understand that the deaf are, in fact, very capable. I firmly believe I can do anything anybody else can do, given the proper training.

Communication would not be as great a barrier if hearing people and deaf people would mutually work toward breaking down the obstacles. I wish the two groups would learn to communicate better with each other.

Tami Saddler:

I agree, John, but whose responsibility is it to assume the leadership role and break down these obstacles? Where do you currently see the efforts being made towards this goal?

Look at the school you went to. Your school placed its emphasis on oral communication. It claimed you would have to struggle to learn to read lips in order to go out and successfully communicate with the hearing world. You were the one who had to make the effort to communicate with the hearing world.

The hearing world does not perceive this lack of communication as their problem. The language/communication barrier is your problem, and it is up to you to break it down. That is the conclusion I come to when I look at who has to make all the effort.

You very seldom find hearing schools teaching their students sign language. They offer classes in French, Spanish, and Latin, but not sign language. Obviously sign language and communicating with the deaf is not a priority. I think this is unfortunate because what are the chances of these students encountering someone who speaks Latin, compared with the chances of meeting someone who is deaf and could greatly benefit from their knowing sign language? Isn't it just as important as learning French or Latin?

I think too frequently in the past the deaf worker has not been hired, not because he lacked the skills for the job, but because the hearing employer feared he would be unable to communicate with the deaf person. Imagine how much the job situation would change if the hearing employer knew sign language! The communication problem would no longer be a factor in determining whether to hire deaf workers. A deaf worker could be hired, promoted, and fired solely on the basis of his ability and job skills.

If sign language was offered to hearing students during their school years it would be a great help to the deaf community. Hearing people would also benefit from the exposure. It would not be a one way street.

The deaf, and organizations serving the deaf, could help promote this by offering to teach sign language classes to various schools and public organizations throughout the country. You have to make it easy for hearing students and adults to be exposed to, and learn this foreign language.

Remember, the hearing world does not perceive it as their problem. They are not going to make any special efforts for the goodness of mankind. They have to be sold on the subject matter as something worth studying, and then it must be offered to them so they can study it without too many hassles.

John Saddler:

Oh, I agree with you, Tami. But I think it is also more complicated than just learning each other's language. It is like a foreign student coming to visit America: he may know the English language by studying it in his own country, but he really doesn't understand America. He doesn't know the American culture. He doesn't know the American system of values.

The same is true of the hearing and deaf worlds. There is a different culture in each of these worlds. There is a lot the hearing world and deaf world need to learn about each other's system of values before they can truly understand each other.

Tina Priest:

I love to dance. I like to go out and enjoy the music. What frustrates me most about being deaf is not being able to really hear the music. I can hear some of the music, but I want to hear all of it! I want to be able to hear a variety of noises, not just some noises. Hearing new and strange noises would be exciting!

Lulu Sinsabaugh:

When I need to communicate with hearing people, I have to write down what I want to say. I am so tired of that! I also get very frustrated trying to lip read what hearing people are saying to me, especially if that person has a beard.

Roxanne Ruiz:

I get frustrated when I miss part of what people are saying to me. I sometimes will miss a single word out of a sentence and that single word changes the entire meaning of the sentence! So I misunderstand a lot of conversations and that frustrates me a lot.

Sometimes I think people talk too fast. Even when they know I am hard of hearing I sometimes think they do that on purpose, so I will not catch what they are saying. I feel like knocking their heads off when they do that! (Laughter.)

Paula Schurz:

When I try to talk to hearing people, they just walk off. When I try to talk with my family, they just nod their heads. Does my family really know what I am saying? Do they really know what I am trying to talk about? If they don't understand, they should let me know.

I also get frustrated because I want to know what they are talking about. Sometimes I understand part of their dialogue, but only rarely do I understand the whole conversation. I feel really left out when my family does not take the time to let me know what topics are being discussed.

Shannon Kidder:

I am most frustrated when I see people use my name without signing. I can't understand what they are saying about me.

Another frustration is when people are talking to me and looking the other way. I can't read their lips if I can't see them.

I also get frustrated when I try to talk with a hearing person and a second hearing person interrupts my conversation. I feel that is so rude! Isn't my conversation just as important as theirs?

Kathy Ferguson:

I can't understand what people are saying to me. Especially on the phone, I only get parts of the conversation. I want to understand everything that is being said.

When my parents are talking with each other or with my brother, I feel left out. I do not understand what they are talking about. I feel I am always behind on the family's news. I think I am always the last person to find out what is going on.

Lori Little:

I am very frustrated when I am working. The hearing workers will tell a joke and laugh, and I have no idea what they are laughing about. I don't understand the office chatter. I want to laugh with them.

I feel left out of my family. If hearing people invite me to a party, frequently, I find myself just sitting there. There is nobody I can communicate with.

I would like to be independent. I wish I could call hearing people on the phone without having to rely on other hearing people to interpret for me.

I hate having to write down things when I want to say something to hearing people, particularly when I am interviewing for a job.

Jenny Simpson:

I wish I could hear beautiful songs!

I don't like it when hearing people feel sorry for me. I am okay, I just can't hear.

Do you trust hearing people?

John Saddler:

I don't classify people. Each person is an individual.

Tami Saddler:

You can trust some hearing people and you can't trust others. The same is true of deaf people: you can trust some and you can't others.

Tina Priest:

It depends. Sometimes it is very hard to tell if you can really trust a person or not. Many times I found out that my hearing friends had made fun of me. Sometimes they would ignore me because I was deaf. They would not care how I felt. Sometimes they would just walk off and leave me standing there alone.

So I don't know how much I trust hearing people.

Lulu Sinsabaugh:

No, sometimes I feel they cheat or fool deaf people. Other times they make the deaf feel irrelevant. Sometimes hearing people hurt my feelings. When deaf people ask for directions, sometimes hearing people will not take the time to make sure they understand the deaf person's questions, and will direct the deaf person to the wrong place.

Paula Schurz:

If they do not show patience with me and my deafness, or obviously do not want to share things with me, then I do not trust them. Even when I know a hearing person pretty well, I will trust him only up to a point, never completely.

Debbie Pruett:

Most of the time I do not trust hearing people, especially hearing people I don't know. I don't like it when I see hearing people make fun of deaf people. I don't like it when hearing people talk behind my back, or use my name without my knowledge or consent.

I can see the expressions of hearing people's faces when they are looking at us. Regardless whether they are talking about me, I can tell when they are talking and making comments about deaf people.

I should say, though, I do trust some hearing people. I know them and they are my friends.

Jenny Simpson:

In some ways I trust them, in other ways I don't. For example, imagine you and I are at a meeting where there are hearing and deaf people. You are hearing and I am deaf. I ask you if you are going to a party later on. You say that you are not. At the same time you tell your hearing friends that you are, in fact, going, but do not to tell the deaf people. I feel that kind of thing happens sometimes.

Do you trust deaf people?

John Saddler:
It depends upon the individual.

Lulu Sinsabaugh:
It depends. Some I trust, others I don't trust. Deaf people can hurt my feelings, too.

Roxanne Ruiz:
Yes, I trust deaf people. I feel they accept me. I am more comfortable with them. True, I have been hurt by deaf people. I do not feel it is by their lying to me. I think the hurt I have felt is due to normal misunderstandings. The basic trust is still there.

Paula Schurz:
So-so. I trust deaf people, but at the same time I am careful in my dealings with them. There are many times when misunderstandings arise.

There are different language levels among the deaf. One deaf person's language level can be so high that another deaf person doesn't really understand what she is talking about. Many deaf people do not understand idioms, so you have to be careful when you use them.

Also, the deaf have a hard time keeping secrets. The rumor mill always seems to be running, which creates a lot of needless misunderstandings and ill feelings towards others in the deaf community.

Shannon Kidder:

Sometimes I trust deaf people, other times I don't. Some deaf people really spread a lot of rumors and don't tell the truth. Deaf people's imaginations can be very active.

Also, keeping a secret is sometimes very hard for a deaf person. Many times I have told a secret to a friend of mine, only to have it spread all over the place!

Debbie Pruett:

Yes and No. I have had friends who were deaf and we trusted each other. Other times, I found out that my deaf friends were just being friendly to see what they could get from me. It is the same as with hearing people: some you can trust, some you can't.

Kathy Ferguson:

It depends upon the person. Deaf people are infamous for spreading rumors. I think the rumors are the result of the deaf world being a small community. Everybody knows everybody else, so there is ample ground for gossip.

I also feel an element of immaturity comes into play with some deaf individuals. Many seem to be stuck in junior high school. There are also a lot of misunderstandings.

Lori Little:

It depends upon the individual. I think the rumor situation is a lot worse for the deaf than the hearing population. The deaf can be very jealous of each other. Deaf people can be very narrow-minded. I think hearing people are more open-minded and are more willing to understand situations. Many deaf people are quick to judge. Deaf people will insult each other very quickly. I think this is mostly due to simple misunderstandings. The deaf can be very selfish. I think this is as a result of the deaf child's not getting enough attention while he is growing up. If he feels neglected by his family because of the deafness, then the child learns to think of himself first - "Nobody else cares for me, so I have to care for myself."

What bothers you the most about hearing people?

John Saddler:

Classification. It frustrates me when hearing people, or any group of people, classify other people or prejudge them. I am an individual and should be judged as an individual. The fact that I am deaf does not mean I have the same abilities or disabilities as all other deaf people.

Classifying people by handicap is the same as labeling a group by nationality or religion. It is frustrating and naive to classify a person, particularly his abilities, because he is a member of a group.

When I meet people, I don't tell them that I'm deaf. I want them to judge me on my abilities. If and when they find out that I'm deaf, that's fine, but first they have had an opportunity to judge the whole me rather than just the deaf part of me.

Tami Saddler:

First, classification. When someone sees a handicapped person, they see the handicap first. Frequently they will not give the handicapped person a chance to show his other qualities and skills. They think "handicapped" and that's it.

Second, people who don't understand the hard of hearing or deaf worlds. Many hearing people think they understand these two worlds, but in reality they don't. What really upsets me is when a hearing person starts telling deaf people what the deaf need. Many times they don't really know what they are talking about. I have seen some hearing teachers in deaf schools do this. They are really good at telling the deaf what is best for them. They may teach the deaf academic subjects, but they really don't understand deafness.

For example; hearing teachers will often say deaf children should always wear their hearing aids. But some deafness is so profound that the hearing aid is more of an irritant than a help. And hearing aids are not all that comfortable. I would suggest that the teacher try wearing a hearing aid for ten hours straight, seven days a week, and see how much he likes it.

Other times they will say that deaf children need to learn how to speak. Some deaf children are just not capable of learning to talk. If the child can't talk, I think it is wrong to force her to talk in the classroom. It can be very embarrassing. Let her be.

I do agree with lip reading training. It is a hearing world and the deaf and hard of hearing will benefit from learning to read lips. It just has to be taught with a bit of common sense and the realization that each deaf person is an individual, and some will be better at it than others.

When I meet people I tell them right away that I am hard of hearing. I am not a very good lip reader so I let them know. I ask them to look directly at me so I have a better chance of understanding what they are saying.

John can frequently get away without telling people he is deaf because he is very good at lip reading. He also has pretty good speech.

John Saddler:

If I am having a problem understanding a person, then I will tell him. I tell him I read lips, and ask him to repeat what he said to me one more time. Usually I get the message.

Tina Priest:

It frustrates me when I am with hearing people and they know I have to read their lips, but they do not face me. When they talk too fast I am lost.

When they do not speak clearly on the phone it really frustrates me. I can not read their lips, so they need to slow down and speak distinctly.

Some hearing people overdo it and that is just as bad. If they yell into the phone or say the words too slowly, then I get just as confused.

Some men's voices are so low, I can't follow what the men are saying. On the other hand, some women's voices are so high I can't follow them either. It is very frustrating.

Lulu Sinsabaugh:

Hearing people give up too easily when trying to communicate with me. When I ask them to repeat what they were saying, they don't want to make the effort or they look really put out.

Another thing that bothers me is the response I often get when I ask a hearing person talking to me to repeat what she has just said. She will often say, "Oh, it's really not very important." If that is true, then why talk to me in the first place? That really bothers me.

Roxanne Ruiz:

I get really frustrated when a hearing person says, "Oh, never mind," when I ask him what he said or, "It is not for you to know," or, "It is not important."

Paula Schurz:

I am annoyed when hearing people know I am in their presence and do not try to include me in their conversations. Even when I am in the same room, they act as though I am not there. They leave me out.

Shannon Kidder:

I don't like it when hearing people make fun of deaf people or sign language.

Sometimes it bothers me when people stare at me when I am signing. I understand they might be interested in deafness, but I don't like it when they stare at me. I think that is rude.

I don't like it when hearing people talk behind my back. I can be in the same room, and they know they can talk without me hearing them. If I am in their presence they should sign, or at least let me know what they are talking about.

Sometimes, when a hearing person talks to me and I don't understand, she will make a strange face. That hurts. I am trying to understand, but the message just isn't getting through.

Debbie Pruett:

It bothers me when hearing people seem to have no patience. Sometimes I don't understand, and I need to ask the speaker to write his message out on a piece of paper. I can tell by the person's expression that he really doesn't want to do that.

I don't like it when hearing people stare at me when I use sign language. It is OK to be curious, but not to stare. That makes me uncomfortable.

Kathy Ferguson:

I don't like it when people make fun of me. I don't like it when they make fun of sign language.

There are times when hearing people avoid me. They know I am there, but they leave me out of their activities and conversations.

Lori Little:

In addition to what Kathy just said, I would add that it bothers me a little when hearing people will ask me stupid questions. For example, "Do you know braille?" What does that have to do with being deaf? Or, "Can you drive a car?" I get tired of answering that one.

Sometimes when I am talking with a hearing person, that person will not give me any feedback as to whether they comprehend what I am saying. Do they really understand me or are they just politely nodding their heads? Why don't they respond in some manner?

I think some hearing people are afraid to stop me when I am talking to them. They are afraid to ask me to explain more clearly what I am trying to say. If they don't understand and they don't tell me, then what is the point of my efforts? They should tell me when they don't understand.

Jenny Simpson:

I get frustrated when hearing people have no patience with deaf people, and when they tell different stories to deaf people than they tell to other people.

When hearing people tell me, "Never mind," after I ask them to repeat what they have just said, I find it really annoying. I should be the one to decide if it is important or not.

What bothers you the most about deaf people?

John Saddler:
Well, the same things that bother me about hearing people: classification and communication. They classify the hearing world as one group. A lot of the deaf claim they don't like the hearing world as a group. They cling stubbornly to their views of hearing people.

Hearing people tune deaf people out because of their handicap. Deaf people tune hearing people out because of their ignorance of deafness. It is sometimes like a civil war. With a little education on both sides, it would not have to be that way.

Tami Saddler:
I don't like all the gossip deaf people spread, but you find that among hearing people also.

Tina Priest:
I really dislike all the rumors they spread. Your so-called friends will stab you in the back at times. Other times, they will waste your time asking really stupid questions when the answer is obvious.

Lulu Sinsabaugh:
Rumors!

Like the hearing, deaf people sometimes don't show patience. They don't want to repeat something they said to someone who missed the message.

The deaf world is small. I think that's why the deaf have to contend with more rumors than the hearing. I get so tired of dealing with rumors. It is also very difficult to keep a secret in the deaf world.

Paula Schurz:

Gossip. A quickness to judge others. Arguing over small things. Misunderstandings; and a seeming reluctance to settle misunderstandings. Sometimes ignoring explanations when they are offered. Though I think these things happen with the hearing population, too, I feel they are more prevalent with the deaf. I believe this happens because of the nature of the handicap. It often leads to misunderstandings, hurt feelings, and emotional responses.

Deaf people have a hard time forgiving each other for things that have happened in the past. We should learn to show more compassion for each other.

Do you trust your parents?

Tami Saddler:

Yes. My mom and dad have always been there for me.

John Saddler:

Yes, I generally trust my parents, but not in everything. I like my independence. I like to find things out for myself. Sometimes what they think and what I think are two different things.

Tami Saddler:

Many young people will doubt what their parents are telling them. I think this is natural, particularly during adolescence. You are growing up and you want your independence. You want to strike out on your own. Even though your parent's advice may be right, you still want to make your own decisions.

The same advice coming from a person other than your parents is more readily acceptable. I think you react this way because this other person does not threaten your independence.

My mom was great. Whenever our family got together, she would take the extra time to make sure I understood everything that was going on. I know some of my deaf friends feel left out of their families, so by the time they are sixteen the reservoir of trust is pretty low.

Roxanne Ruiz:

That is a really, good, tough question. In some ways yes. I know they try hard to help me understand what they really mean. I know they had a hard time raising me. At times it is hard to communicate with them.

My parents did not learn sign language. They would make gestures. They know they have to talk loud in order for me to understand. Most of the time this is fine, I can understand what they are saying to me. I trust them, but the communication is hard sometimes and misunderstandings do occur.

Paula Schurz:

Sure. Sometimes, though, I don't understand why they don't tell me about what is happening with the other members of my family. They tell my brother and sister, but why not me? Why am I always the last person to hear the news?

Shannon Kidder:

Medium. Sometimes I talk with my mom or my dad. I will tell them a story and ask them not to tell anybody else. Then they would go and tell my sisters. I really don't like that. In the past this happened all the time. It is getting better now, as they realize how much this upsets me. I do feel that my parents always tell me the truth.

Debbie Pruett:

Most of the time I try to trust them, but sometimes I do not feel I can. Though I have had many frustrations with my family, I still love them.

For example, I have a hearing sister. Many times she and my mother would talk without using sign language. I felt very left out and suspicious of what they were talking about. I wish my parents would sign everything so that I would not be left out.

Other times, I would want to talk with my mom. Just as I would be starting our conversation, my sister would interrupt and take my mom's attention away. This really frustrated me.

I ask parents of deaf children to please learn sign language so that their children will not feel left out. It would also be of great help if the other siblings would learn and use sign language. Then the whole family would be able to talk with each other.

Lori Little:

No. They would not communicate with me. I feel they do not tell me the truth. They never advise me.

I remember one time my grandmother gave me two thousand dollars for Christmas. My father said it had been invested for me. When I was a senior in high school, I applied for financial assistance. The loan application asked how much money I had in the bank. I wrote down two thousand dollars. Well, that was too much money so they turned down my request.

Shortly after that, I was curious to know just how much money I did have in the bank. I asked my mom exactly how much money I had in my saving account. When she said none, I was shocked. I asked her where the money I had been given was. She said it had been used to purchase a car for me. It was true I had received a car from my parents, but I hadn't been told that the "gift" was bought with my money! They had never taken the time to explain that to me, or even to ask if I wanted to use the money for that purpose. So first I was not granted financial assistance because I thought I had money, and then I found out that I didn't really have it!

When it comes to family matters, I am always behind on the news. My parents never inform me. I always have to ask them what is going on.

What do you fear the most?

John Saddler:
   God! (Laughter.)

Tami Saddler:
   My biggest fear is losing all my hearing. I don't know how
to read lips without the help of what hearing I do have. Currently, I am able to combine what I hear with some lip reading and understand most conversations.
   I have lost eighty percent of my hearing in one ear and about
seventy percent in the other ear. Even so, I can understand
most conversations with people who have a voice of medium
pitch. But it gets really difficult if the person has a high, soft
voice, or if I am in a room with a lot of other noises. Sometimes
my hearing is really funny. I can not hear the telephone ring,
but I can hear the air conditioner click on and off. There are
certain sounds I can pick out very well and there are others I
do not hear at all. If I am familiar with a sound, then it is easier
for me to anticipate its frequency and be ready for it. If the
room is really quiet it is surprising how much I can pick up.
   I can imagine it must be very frustrating for a hearing person to be around someone who is hard of hearing. Sometimes they seem to hear just fine and other times there is no
response at all. What is wrong with them? Why are they
ignoring me when I address them? Are they stuck-up? Why
can they hear me sometimes and then not at other times?
That is the nature of being hard of hearing, at least in my
case. There seems to be no set pattern in my ability to hear.
That leads to frustrations for both hearing people and for me.
   Getting back to your question, if I woke up some morning
and found out that I was no longer able to hear at all, I'm

afraid I would be totally lost. The doctors have told me that this is a very real possibility and it scares me. Though I have no problem using sign language and joining the deaf world, I do not want to leave the hearing world. It is where I have spent most of my life.

John Saddler:

Tami is hard of hearing and I understand her fears. I think she would find the deaf world more difficult. There are a lot of gaps in your education if you are deaf. In order to success-fully compete with the hearing world, you have to work doubly hard to catch up and fill these gaps.

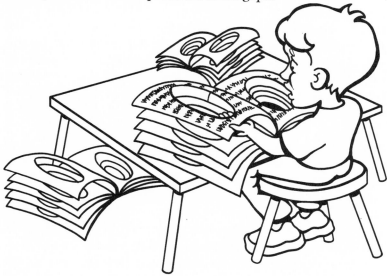

If I really had a choice, I would rather be hard of hearing than profoundly deaf. Though the hard of hearing are fre-quently stuck in a never-never land between the hearing and deaf worlds, I would still like to be able to hear some music.

Roxanne Ruiz:

I think what scares me the most is being stuck in the hearing world. It is hard for me to catch what they are saying. I am not really comfortable being with them. There is really no way for me to fit in.

Sometimes I get scared that the deaf will think I hear too much or speak too well and reject me. My deaf friends like me a lot and I like them. I am happy to interpret for them, but sometimes I do not show how much I can hear or how well I can speak, because I don't want them to think I am showing off. I do not want them to reject me. I don't want to be alone.

Debbie Pruett:

The cops! (Laughter.) I imagine that I am stopped by the police for speeding or something. I can't hear them and try to get out my driver's license. I don't want them to think I am pulling out a gun and then shoot me.

Kathy Ferguson:

Being alone and not being able to hear someone break into my house.

Lori Little:

If I got married to a deaf man and my children were deaf, would my brothers, sisters, mother and father accept us? Or would they ignore us because we were deaf? Would they invite us over for Christmas? Even if they did, would they ignore us and give their attention to the other hearing relatives? I do not want to lose my family. I want to be close to them.

Do you wear a hearing aid? Do you like it? Does it help?

Tami Saddler:

At work I wear one, but not at home or with my family. When I am at home or with my family I use total communication. I have some hearing, but when the person I am with uses signs, I am able to communicate without the use of the hearing aid.

I like the hearing aid when I need to use the telephone, and when I listen to the radio. But I hate it when I am in the room with a lot of other people. I hate it when I am in a room where there is a lot of typing. It gives me a headache.

John Saddler:

I do not wear a hearing aid at all. I am profoundly deaf and it doesn't do me any good. I wish I could benefit from one.

Tina Priest:

Yes, I wear one. It helps me. I like it. When I am alone or with my deaf friends I will not wear it. When I know I will be with hearing people or have to talk on the phone, then I put it on.

It really doesn't bother me unless I have an old, ill fitting ear mold. Then it whistles a lot.[25] I guess the only other time

---

[25]Hearing aids must be custom fitted with proper hearing aid ear molds. When the ear mold does not perfectly conform to the shape of the ear canal of the user, or is not properly placed in the ear, "feedback" will often occur. It is very high pitched and sounds like a steady whistle. This is because the microphone of the hearing aid is in such close proximity to the output of the device. This is the same annoying feedback that sometimes occurs in microphones, when the amplification of the background noise is over-boosted.

that it really bothers me is when I have an ear infection. Then it really hurts.

Without my hearing aid, I feel very much in the deaf world. When I have it on, I feel I am half in the deaf world and half in the hard of hearing world.

Roxanne Ruiz:

No, I don't wear one. I don't like using one because it makes more noise than anything else. It makes it harder for me to hear you because it makes all the other noises around me louder.

Paula Schurz:

Yes, I always wear one hearing aid. It helps me a lot. I am really quite uncomfortable when I am not wearing my hearing aid. I do not like hearing nothing.

I especially want to be able to hear my son if he starts to cry. When my hearing aid is not on or working properly, I feel I have to be very alert with my eyes, continuously checking around me so that I don't miss anything. That can be very tiring.

Even with my hearing aid on, I still have a hard time understanding people with high pitched voices. I also have a hard time understanding little children's voices because they talk so softly.

Shannon Kidder:

Yes, I wear two hearing aids. I wear them all the time unless I have an ear infection.

Kathy Ferguson:

Yes, I wear two hearing aids. I feel they help me a lot. I really want both of them on all the time. I think the two together help my balance. Without the hearing aids, I can not hear the telephone or the doorbell.

Jenny Simpson:

No, I do not wear a hearing aid now. I have in the past. I wore a "body aid"[26] until I was about ten years old. When I was thirteen I got a behind-the-ear hearing aid, but I didn't use it very much. Now I don't use one at all.

I don't like wearing one because I know it sometimes whistles and I hate to bother people. I have repeatedly had new ear molds made but it still whistled so I decided to forget it.

---

[26]A "body aid" refers to a very powerful hearing aid that is the size of a man's shirt pocket. Its most common use is with young children who are severely/profoundly hearing impaired.

Frequently it also functions as miniature FM receiver/amplifier for these children. The classroom teacher will use it in conjunction with an FM transmitter to direct his or her speech directly to this amplifying device worn by the children. Only the FM voice of the teacher is received and amplified. In this way all other distracting noises in the classroom can be shut out.

At the onset of adolescence most hearing impaired individuals switch to smaller, less conspicuous aids. These are usually "behind the ear" or "all in the ear" styled instruments. They are not as powerful, and do not have the FM features or the fidelity of the "body aids."

Do you believe in oral communication programs for teaching deaf children?

Tami Saddler:
  Yes, one hundred percent.

John Saddler:
  Yes, but I believe such programs should be coupled with signs. The English language should not only be spoken with the mouth, but also with the hands.

Tina Priest:
  It depends upon how well the child can hear. I would start the child in an oral program to encourage his speech development, but if the child was not responding, then I would quickly introduce sign language. If the child is born profoundly deaf then I would use sign language immediately.

Roxanne Ruiz:
  I do not believe in a strictly oral approach. I think it is better to have both signs and oral instruction. I think if the deaf can not use signs in their education then they lose a lot of enthusiasm for learning. It is too frustrating for them.
  I think, though, that it is a good idea for a child to have good oral instruction so that in the future she will be able to communicate with hearing people.

Paula Schurz:
  No. It is too hard to try to understand what teachers are saying just by reading their lips. Too many words look alike. Too many words sound similar. Speech and communication

that is backed up with signing is so much clearer and easier to understand.

Having said that, I do feel it is important for children to have a good enthusiastic program in speech development. That will give them the opportunity to develop their speech to the point where they will be able to communicate with hearing children. Good communication enriches the sharing/socialization process of people.

Shannon Kidder:

I believe in it to some degree. It depends upon the feeling of the child. If the child is comfortable and making progress in an oral program, then fine.

Personally, since I am deaf, I would want my own children to learn sign language so that I could communicate with them. I would not want situations in which they do not understand what I am trying to tell them. I also don't want situations where I don't understand what they are trying to tell me.

Kathy Ferguson:

No. Deaf children are more comfortable if they are permitted to use signs. There is too much frustration in trying to rely on speech and lip reading alone. We do not force hearing people to use only signs. Why is it that some hearing people think it is right to force deaf people to use only speech?

Lori Little:

I am against an oral approach. Some hearing teachers do try to force some deaf students to do without signs. They will

even slap the deaf children's hands if they catch them signing. I think this is mean. Deaf children don't learn very much
under these conditions. Their vocabulary is very limited.

When I went to an oral school I felt it was a big waste of
time. I didn't learn very much. I later transferred to a school
that taught using both signs and speech and I learned a lot
more.

Jenny Simpson:

No! Period! For one reason or another, many deaf people
do not acquire good oral communication skills. They cannot help it. Then when they are forced to try to communicate with other people without sign language they are very
frustrated.

Deaf people have a right to learn sign language. Who has
the right to say the deaf cannot communicate in this manner?

I know when several of my college friends first arrived
here they had only oral communication skills. They were
shocked when they saw other students using sign language.
Some of them had been so isolated that they didn't even
know sign language existed! But they very quickly picked it
up and are now much happier. Life is so much easier for
them. Communication is no longer such a struggle.

Do you prefer signing in English or American Sign Language?

Tami Saddler:

Both have their place. Signed English is used for school and learning the English language. ASL is used in the deaf culture, and the deaf have a right to use their own language. Why shouldn't the deaf be able use the language of their choice when they are with each other?

ASL involves communication using concepts. Therefore, it is a lot faster than Signed English. If the important thing is to get the concept across, why make it any harder than necessary?

I do feel that ASL alone would not be a good idea. If a child was raised by deaf parents who only exposed the child to ASL and the child's school only used ASL, then I think she would have a major problem when she attempted to learn the English language. This would be especially true when communication involved hearing people who are, of course, only familiar with English.

John Saddler:

I prefer Signed English. I believe Signed English has a stronger vocabulary structure than ASL. ASL only defines the object with pictures and gestures.

Tina Priest:

I associate with both hard of hearing and deaf people. With both groups I see a mixture of Signed English and ASL. Sometimes this is called PSE, Pidgin Signed English.

Watching Signed English alone is very boring. It makes you want to go to sleep.

For young deaf children, I would recommend SEE, Signing Exact English. This will be most beneficial for them in learning the English language. When they are older, they can be introduced to ASL.

Lulu Sinsabaugh:

I like both. Which I use depends upon who I am with. If the other person is using English, then I will sign in English. If the other person uses ASL, then I will sign in ASL. Given the choice, I prefer ASL because it is a lot faster.

Paula Schurz:

I use ASL. Even though my mind thinks in English, I sign in ASL because it is faster. Only about ten percent of the deaf adults I know use Signed English.

Shannon Kidder:

I prefer Signed English. I am more used to it. When I use ASL it is harder for me to write proper English.

Debbie Pruett:

I prefer Signed English. I feel more comfortable when my writing and signing have the same structure. Also, it is easier for me to communicate with hearing people when I use English. Hearing people that use sign language use the English language for their structure. They have a hard time understanding me if I use ASL. When I am communicating with my deaf friends, I will frequently end up using a mixture of Signed English and ASL.

Lori Little:

I prefer ASL. ASL is faster, needing fewer signs for the same concept. It is a lot more enjoyable. When I use Signed English I fall asleep.

What special devices do you like most in your home?

Tami Saddler:

We have a TDD, a special light that blinks on and off when the telephone rings, and an alarm clock light that wakes me up in morning. Since my hearing has decreased, I can't hear the telephone at times or the noise of a regular alarm clock.

John Saddler:

We also have a closed-captioner for our TV. Of all our devices, I like that one the most.

Tami Saddler:

We don't even go to regular movie theaters. We would miss too much of the dialogue. We just wait until the movie comes out on video tape. We look for the symbol on the box telling us it has been closed captioned and then rent it. Today, almost all the movies are closed captioned.

Tina Priest:

I have a closed captioner, a TTY,[27] and a light for the phone. I need to get a light for the doorbell. I know there have been times when people have knocked on the door and have rung the doorbell and I have not heard them.

---

[27]A TTY is an early version of what was previously described as a TTD, a machine enabling deaf people to communicate using the telephone. They function in the same basic manner and for the same purpose. Early TTYs were very large machines and have generally been replaced by TDDs that are the size of small portable typewriters.

Lulu Sinsabaugh:

We have a TDD, a closed-captioner, a light for the door-bell, a light for the phone, a baby-crier,[28] and a bed vibrator connected to my alarm clock.

In the past I tried a light for my alarm. Sometimes I would be in such a deep sleep that I would not wake up when the light went on. So to be safe, now I have the bed vibrator alarm.

---

[28]A baby-crier is a device that will flash a light on and off in one room in response to the noise generated in another room. It is frequently used by deaf parents to monitor the sounds of their newborn.

Would you raise a deaf child in the same way that you were raised by your parents?

John Saddler:

No! I would raise my child differently. I don't think my parents knew how to raise me. Most of the time my parents left me out. They did not teach me about the world. They didn't help me learn the English language. When I became deaf at five years of age they were lost.

I firmly believe it is the parents' responsibility to develop the deaf child's aptitudes. Parents have to be teachers to their children, particularly if the children are deaf! That is what I would do differently: I would take the time to educate my child.

If I could, I would teach my deaf child sign language while he was still in the womb! I would teach him English. I would even try to develop his speaking skills! (laughter)

Tami Saddler:

I don't think I would spoil the child as I was. I would not want to the child to think she was too special. That can lead to problems.

I think my mother and father believed they were responsible for my deafness, so they tried to compensate by spoiling me. I am the baby of the family and I think they let me get away with too much and bought me too many things.

On the other hand, my parents were good teachers. Whenever my mom heard me pronounce a word wrong she would work with me right then to make sure I pronounced it correctly. Even when I was a young girl she did that, before we all realized I had a hearing problem. She also did that with my brothers. She made a point of helping us speak correctly and made sure that we knew the meaning of the words we were using.

I remember coming home and telling her we had learned all about "Hamburger Lincoln" in school. My mom said, "Who?" I said, "You know, Mom, the President!" She said, "Oh, Tami, you mean *Abraham* Lincoln!" That happened when I was in first grade.

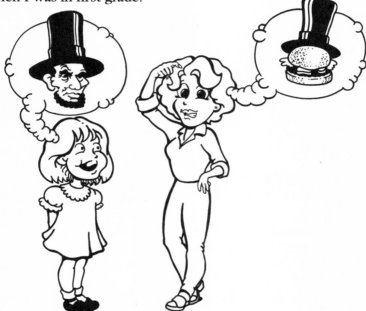

John Saddler:

I would like to accelerate my child's education as much as I could. I would like to get him into college when he is thirteen!

I know this would put him in a different situation. The students in his classes would be about ten years older, but I think it would help him a lot. He would know so much more. He would be more aware at a young age. He would be much more prepared to deal with the world.

I am not saying this could always be done, but it is possible! Oh, I guess what I am saying, is that I would push him as far as I could. I would do everything possible to further his education.

Tami Saddler:

I think that is nuts. If you put a kid into college at the age of thirteen, he is going to be too confused. He might be a lot smarter, but he is never going to have a chance to be a kid!

I think during the teenage years, after homework is done, a child should be able to develop socially with his friends. There is no way that this social development is going to occur for a thirteen year old with classmates who are ten years his senior! I would never put my child in college at that age!

John Saddler:

Well, I agree with a lot of what Tami is saying. I just do not want to limit the child's education. I have seen that done too often with deaf children.

Tina Priest:

If I had a deaf child, I guess I would raise him the same way I was raised. My mom learned sign language when I was very young. We communicated a lot and I have stayed very close to her. My father did not learn sign language, so I did not talk with him very much. I am not as close to my father.

Lulu Sinsabaugh:

No, I had a hard life with my parents. I would do it differently. First of all, I would sign with my child. My parents really did not sign and it was very difficult. I would give my child a lot stronger support for learning. I would make sure my child was not involved in drugs. I would do what I could to insure he associated with good groups.

Roxanne Ruiz:

No, I would use sign language with my child. My parents are not bad, but they communicate as the hearing world communicates, using their voices. That is fine for them, but it is very difficult for me. I would use my voice, too, but I would definitely support it with sign language. I understand my parents were very busy, but I would like to think I could spend more time teaching my deaf child. Deaf children need more instruction because they miss so much.

Paula Schurz:

I would do two things differently. First, I would use sign language with my child. That would open up communication between us. Secondly, I would do those activities that would show and reinforce to him that he is important to me and to the family. I would strive to include him in all the family activities. I would not leave him out of conversations. I would try to be conscious of situations where he might feel lonely.

Debbie Pruett:

No, I would allow my child to learn about deafness. I would insure that we as a family accepted him and his deafness. We would all know sign language.

My father never learned sign language. He was never comfortable when I had my deaf friends come to our house, and my deaf friends could feel that. They never talked with my father and did not feel welcome.

Because my family does not know sign language other than simple gestures like those for "time" and "eat," and doesn't make the effort to communicate with me, I'm more comfortable talking with my deaf friends than with my own family. For example, at dinner my family talks and I can't understand what they are saying. I just eat. When I want to talk with someone I go outside of my family.

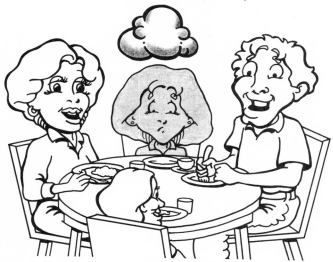

My father works on cars a lot. When I feel my car has a problem, I ask him to check it out. Sometimes there is actually a problem and at other times he tells me it is nothing. I can tell my father gets frustrated with me when there is nothing wrong with the car.

I wish I could ask him to teach me about cars. That way I could check the car out myself and not bother him. But we don't communicate. He doesn't know sign language and doesn't take time to be with me.

I am closest to my Aunt Peg. She realizes that I am deaf and understands I am left out. She takes the time to tell me what is happening in my family.

Just this past year, I finally got to know my sister. When we were growing up, we were constantly fighting. Just recently we had a good sister-to-sister talk. She told me that while we were growing up, she defended me whenever someone would make fun of me because I was deaf. I never knew that! All of these years we never communicated. Now, finally, we are beginning to take the time to talk to each other.

What would I do differently with my child? I would accept his deafness. I would use sign language. I would take the time to communicate with him, and I would allow him to be a part of the deaf world.

Kathy Ferguson:

I would do pretty much the same as my parents did with me. I wish my father had learned sign language when I was a young girl. My mother learned sign language years ago, but it was only last year that my father took a class. Many years went by before I was able to talk with him. When my deaf friends would come over to the house, my father was left out. If only he had known sign language he could have talked with them. I would have liked that.

If I married a man who did not know sign language, I would encourage him to learn it. I feel it is important for both parents to be able to talk with their children.

Lori Little:

No, I would do things a lot differently! First, I would make the effort to communicate with my child. I would learn sign language. I would want my husband to learn sign language. With sign language there is no excuse for not communicating with your child. It solves a lot of problems.

While I was growing up my parents did not know sign language. When my father wanted to talk with me, he would type the message out on my TTY. Then I would have to type my response back to him. This was very interesting when we had arguments!

My parents could communicate with my hearing sister, but there was no communication with me. I don't think this was fair. My sister could always create a story or blame something on me, and I had no means of defending myself. Who could I talk to about my problems or feelings? There was nobody.

Secondly, I would teach my child to be proud. Deafness doesn't mean stupidity. I remember one summer during my high school years, I wanted to work at a car wash to earn extra money. My mom refused to let me because she didn't want other people to think I was stupid. I was denied a work experience because she was concerned about what other people would think! I don't agree with that at all. I would let my child have work experiences while she was growing up. It builds self-concept and pride.

Jenny Simpson:
I would take more time with my deaf child to explain things to her, particularly if I was disciplining her. I remember being sent to my room because I had done something wrong. Too many times I really didn't know why I was being punished.

My mom was pretty good. She learned sign language. She taught me manners. She took the time to explain a lot about the world to me.

Did your mother and father accept your deafness equally?

Tina Priest:

Yes, even though my father did not learn sign language, I feel he accepted my deafness. If I didn't understand what he said to me, he would repeat it. He was very patient.

Lulu Sinsabaugh:

I think they accepted my being deaf, but they still did not treat me right. They didn't learn sign language. I think that was more a result of being lazy than of not accepting my deafness.

Roxanne Ruiz:

Yes, I think they accepted my deafness. It is a part of me, and I feel they accept that.

Paula Schurz:

Yes. Both my parents accepted my deafness equally. I didn't learn sign language until I was twelve. I asked them at that time if they wanted to learn sign language, and they both said no. I don't think this was a symptom of not accepting my deafness. I think they were a little afraid of sign language. I think they thought it would prevent me from developing my speech.

Although I can understand that, it would have been a lot easier for me if they had learned sign language. We are reasonably successful in communicating verbally, but there are many times we have to write down what we want to say to each other.

If they had learned sign language, they would have been able to communicate with my deaf friends when they came over to the house. As things turned out, I had to act as an interpreter or my parents would have to write things down. Such situations are not conducive to getting to know your children's friends!

Debbie Pruett:

I think my mother accepted my deafness, but she didn't learn sign language. My father really did not know how to deal with my deafness. He had two daughters, one hearing and one deaf. He just didn't know how to deal with me. I think one reason he refused to learn sign language is that he thought he could force me to be more like a hearing person.

I want to be close to my father. I would like to be closer to my mother, too. But that takes real communication and we just don't have it. If they would learn sign language it would really help. I wish they would have done that while I was growing up.

Lori Little:

They both had a very hard time accepting my deafness. Even today, I still feel they do not completely accept it.

Just last winter, my father told me he wished he had learned sign language years ago. So I do see some movement towards acceptance, at least on his part.

Jenny Simpson:

I think my mother accepted it more than my father. My mother learned sign language when I was very young. My father never made that effort.

Who helped you more, your mother or your father?

John Saddler:
   My mother. She was always there for me.
   My father had to work two jobs, so his time was very limited.

Tami Saddler:
   My mother. She was always telling me there were no limitations just because I was deaf. I could do anything I wanted to if I put my mind to it.
   My father took a different view. He thought if you had a hearing problem, you had a lot of limitations. He had all these reasons why I couldn't do something. I remember him telling me I couldn't do a particular job because it required me to hear a beeper. That was nonsense. I got the job and had no problem. Even if you can't hear the beeper when it beeps, you can feel it.
   I agree there are some limitations. For instance, if you were profoundly deaf, I think you would have a tough time handling the phone as a sales representative. I think it would be tough being a doctor because you couldn't hear the patients' problems. I don't see how you could be an airline pilot, and I don't believe the Armed Forces have much demand for deaf soldiers. There are some limitations, but that doesn't mean there are not a whole lot of opportunities available to the motivated individual. You can't let some limitations become an excuse for not being creative.

Lulu Sinsabaugh:
   Neither one of them! Well...my mom did help at times by finger-spelling those things she thought I should understand.

And my dad did help me from time to time with my homework.

Roxanne Ruiz:

My father helps me the most. He wants me to be good at things. He teaches me a lot about sports; he helps me with my school work. My mother helps me, too, when I need to buy clothes or to share "girl talk"; but my father helps me the most.

Paula Schurz:

Mostly my mom. She worked with me on my speech. I am closer to my mom because of the time we spent together. My dad tries to teach me about life. He tries to prepare me so I won't be taken for a sucker in various situations. He knows a lot about cars and is always helping me when I have car problems.

Were your brothers and sisters jealous of the attention your parents gave you because of your deafness?

John Saddler:
No, because my parents didn't treat me any differently.

Tami Saddler:
No, but my father did treat me differently than my brother. My father is a little old-fashioned, and he expects a lot more from my brother because he is a male.

By the time I had started losing my hearing, my brother had already moved out of the house; so the extra attention I received from the deafness occurred too late to be a factor in sibling rivalry.

Lulu Sinsabaugh:
I don't think my hearing sister was jealous because of the attention I got from my parents. My parents gave her more attention than they gave me or my other hard of hearing sisters! I think that was because it was easier to communicate with her. They had never learned sign language. I know my hard of hearing sisters were never jealous of me.

One time my hearing sister told me that she wished she were deaf. Then she would then be able to ignore the yelling and screaming in the household, just like me. But I think she was just saying that in a moment of exasperation!

Paula Schurz:
No, I don't think there were jealousies on the part of my siblings because of my deafness. I think a lot of conflicts

arose because I was the oldest and I didn't like taking suggestions from my younger sister and brother.

My deafness put me at a disadvantage when it came to knowing what was going on with the family. Many times I felt left out of the news or the family plans. That made it more difficult for me to hold my own with my siblings.

When you were growing up, did you have any problems with the hearing children in your neighborhood?

John Saddler:

I grew up with hearing people. I was never with other deaf children. The hearing kids treated me differently because they knew I was deaf. Many times, when it was time to pick teams to play a game, I would be the last one picked.

Tami Saddler:

That also happened to me a lot. I was usually the last one picked. I don't know if it was because of my hearing, or if I was just not that good a player.

Remember the game "Red Rover"? Two teams would line up facing each other and then call out, "Red Rover, Red Rover, send _____ over"! Then the person whose name was called would run over to the other line and try to break through it. Well, they never called my name, or if they did I never heard it!

If it was a girls team, there would be times I would be picked. I was pretty well accepted by the girls' groups, but when it came to co-ed games it was a different story.

All in all, I felt pretty popular and generally accepted until eighth grade. Then my hearing loss became quite severe, and I had real problems. My hearing friends thought I was day-dreaming. They thought I wasn't paying attention. Some thought I was on drugs. I was losing my ability to communicate with them.

I started withdrawing because I couldn't understand what was going on. The slumber parties that used to be so much fun were now pretty boring. Many of my friends started to think I was stuck up because I didn't respond to them. I remember several kids wanted to beat me up because of that.

Perhaps a part of this was my fault because at that time I was not willing to accept the fact that I had a hearing problem. I didn't want to admit it, so I didn't tell anyone. I guess that was not fair to my friends. I should have told them.

When I transferred to a school for the deaf, I lost what little remaining contact I had. When I arrived at the deaf school I didn't know a soul. I didn't know sign language. I couldn't communicate. A lot of the deaf students felt my hearing and my speech were too good, so they didn't accept me. Let me tell you, I was one lonely teenager!

Even now, I really have only two hearing friends. One of them is an interpreter and the other is actually hard of hearing. I don't socialize with hearing people like I used to. It is too frustrating. At the same time, I know I am only a visitor to the deaf world. I am hard of hearing and really don't belong there either.

John does not socialize in the deaf world either. Even though he is profoundly deaf, he was raised in hearing schools without sign language. His vocabulary and language level is very high. He also has pretty good speech. Because of this, most deaf people do not feel comfortable with him.

I think John is an example of another, separate group of individuals: those who are deaf, but were raised in an oral environment and whose education is more or less on par with their hearing contemporaries. These groups visit each other's worlds, but they really are not the same: there are the hearing, the hard of hearing, the deaf, and finally, the oral deaf, who are so well educated that they frequently do not relate with the other deaf.

Tina Priest:

When I was young, most of the neighborhood kids would play with me. Some would not and would leave me alone. I don't remember any of them making fun of me.

When I was a little older, I think some of the hearing kids in my neighborhood liked to get me into trouble. They would influence me to do the wrong thing. My mother would try to tell me not to go with them, but I didn't always listen.

Lulu Sinsabaugh:

Yes, they made fun of me because I couldn't hear. I remember they would laugh at the bus I rode on. They knew it was a special bus because it had the name of our school on it. Most of the time, I would just stay at home. I didn't go outside to play.

Paula Schurz:

Sometimes I would follow my brother or sister when they went out in the neighborhood. I would play with their friends or go swimming with them. But most of the time, I would just stay at home.

Shannon Kidder:

I had no problem playing with my hearing friends. We would use our own sign language. Other times I could read their lips pretty well.

Debbie Pruett:

Yes, there were problems. Some of the kids would make fun of my deafness. Some of the parents and kids would tell other people not to play with me because I was deaf and dumb. Other kids were fine. Some of them learned sign language to communicate with me.

As I got older, some of the kids would try to influence me to get involved with smoking and drugs. They introduced me to both of these things.

I remember them asking me if I smoked and then saying, "Why not try it?" I thought of my parents: they smoked, so I figured it couldn't be that bad for you. So I started smoking with the neighborhood kids. I also tried some drugs with them. I don't do that anymore.

I wish my parents had talked with me more about what is good and what is bad for you. Because they didn't spend time with me, I ended up spending my time with the neighborhood group. I see now that their influence was not always good.

Lori Little:

Sometimes they would blame me for something that would go wrong. Sometimes they would leave me out of their games. It was very frustrating. I wanted to have friends but did not feel that they really accepted me.

Jenny Simpson:

No, I had no problems. Some of the neighborhood kids even learned sign language to communicate with me.

When I was a freshman in high school, I remember seeing some hearing kids laughing and making funny signs at me and my fellow students as we rode the bus to school. The bus had the name of our school on the outside of it so they knew we were deaf. But other than that, I had no problems.

Did you like the schools you went to?

Tami Saddler:
I didn't like the hearing schools because they didn't teach me enough. They didn't teach me the basics. The teachers didn't know I had a hearing problem. They thought I was daydreaming. Naturally, they spent their time with the students who paid attention.

During the parent/teacher conferences, my mom told the teachers that I had a hearing problem, that I should sit in the front row of the classes, and that I needed individual attention. They never acted on that information.

I graduated from eighth grade with straight 5's. That means I got an F in every subject. The principal, who didn't know I had a hearing problem, agreed to let me graduate under the condition that I would attend summer school.

He later fired two of my teachers. I don't know if it was because of the way they handled my situation. I do know they had not reported my problems to the office and they had not given me the attention I needed.

I liked the deaf school because I got the individual attention I needed. I didn't know things I should have learned in elementary and junior high. I learned these while I attended the deaf high school.

I do feel, though, that the deaf school I went to was behind. What they were teaching in high school, I had already seen in the regular sixth, seventh, and eighth grades. A normal high school should be teaching beyond the basics. I am afraid the students graduating from that school will be lost when they get to college.

But for my situation, it was great.

John Saddler:
Yes, I liked the schools, but I wish I had interpreters in the classes.

Paula Schurz:
Academically, I preferred the hearing school. It moved faster and was more advanced. For the socialization and friendships I established, I preferred the deaf school.

Shannon Kidder:
I was a little frustrated with the school I went to. Sometimes it was too easy for me.

Lori Little:
Though I only went there for my senior year in high school, I liked the deaf school I attended in Tucson. There were a lot of clubs and activities to get involved with. I met a lot of friends in these clubs. I also enjoyed the independence I experienced there.

I would consider sending my own deaf children to a residential school during their high school years. I would give them that option. I think in the deaf school they would have more opportunities to join clubs and be a part of school activities.

Though my first inclination would be to send them to a deaf school, I would certainly allow them to go a regular high school if they wanted to and could manage there. Where are they going to experience the greatest growth and be the most comfortable?

I would not, though, want to send my child to a residential school while she was young, especially if that would mean sending her far from home. If it was a choice between sending her to a regular school or a residential school, I would probably move the family to the town where the residential school was located, so she could attend as a day student.

Do you remember any favorite teachers? Why were they your favorites?

John Saddler:

Yes, I had a favorite elementary teacher. She spent a lot of time with me.

I had a science teacher I really liked. He was very patient with me. He would go over and over a point to make sure I understood the concept.

My favorite teacher in high school let me go as fast as I could. He gave me a lot of individual freedom to progress though the material as rapidly as possible. I was a self-starter and very motivated. I liked him because he encouraged me and did not hold me back.

I did not participate in many of the classroom discussions because I could not follow them. I wish I'd had an interpreter during those years.

Tami Saddler:

I don't remember any in elementary school that I were my favorites, but I had two in high school. One was my English teacher. She told me that I wasn't stupid. She told me I had the potential to become a writer.

The other one was my math teacher. He also told me I wasn't stupid - lazy maybe, but not stupid! Both of them helped build up my confidence. I really needed that reassurance at that time in my life.

You know, I flunked that math teachers's algebra class. The deaf school told me that I had to stay another year in school because of that. I wish other teachers had been that honest with their grades instead of just passing me.

My senior year in high school, I graduated with all A's and B's, except for one C. I received a scholarship and a creative writing award. It was all because these two people gave me confidence in myself.

Tina Priest:

I had a favorite elementary teacher. She not only taught the subject matter, but also taught us a lot about what was going on in life. She was a humorous teacher. She would makes us all laugh.

My favorite high school teacher was my reading teacher. He would always challenge me to do things better. Even if I got a 97% on an exam, he would encourage me to shoot for a 100% the next time.

Roxanne Ruiz:

I had a lot of favorite elementary teachers. They showed me a lot of attention and gave me a lot of help.

In high school, I have one favorite teacher. She is my reading and English teacher. She gives me the same kind of attention I received in the elementary grades. She is like a mother to me. She teaches me about a lot of things. She cares about me. She encourages me. She doesn't waste any of the class time. She teaches the whole period.

Paula Schurz:

In public school, I had an elementary school teacher that taught me in a way that I could easily understand. She was patient with me. She gave me a lot of individual attention.

In high school I had two teachers I really liked. One, a deaf teacher, would talk about the deaf culture. I liked learning about that.

The other was one of my math teachers. He would not waste our time and taught a new lesson every day. He would also teach us how math could be applied to money matters in real life.

Shannon Kidder:

In fourth grade I had a teacher that really had a lot of enthusiasm. She really made learning exciting. She taught math and English. She always used lots of examples for the things she was teaching us.

She was always challenging us in different ways. In math we had a lot of games. In English she would encourage us to write stories. She always had class projects for us such as hatching chicken eggs.

In high school, I had a really enthusiastic reading teacher. This teacher would have us read a book and then write about it. I learned a lot.

Another favorite was my chemistry teacher. I learned a lot of vocabulary from him. He never wasted my time. He would relate how chemistry applied to the real world. I liked that.

Debbie Pruett:

I didn't have a favorite in elementary school. In junior high school, I had a language teacher I really liked. I learned a lot from her. She would have the deaf kids come to her house all the time to swim in her pool. We felt we were in a big family with her. I had a favorite high school teacher. She taught English. She was always helpful in correcting my language. She showed a lot of patience with me. She never gave up on us.

Lori Little:

In fifth grade I had a teacher that taught reading and history. She really motivated the students with good examples.

She asked the students for their opinions. There was a free exchange of ideas in her classroom.

In high school, I had two favorites. One was a hearing woman who taught English. She was strict and demanded that I do my best.

The other was a deaf man who taught philosophy. He was very skilled in sign language and was fascinating to watch. His lectures were never boring. He would have guest speakers come into the classroom and present their ideas. He encouraged us to learn and explore new ideas.

Do you remember any teachers that you thought were not very good?

John Saddler:

I think all my teachers were pretty good.

Tami Saddler:

Well, my elementary teachers were not that good. They kept passing me on the next higher grade, even though I wasn't mastering the material in their classes. Even worse were my junior high school teachers. Though they knew I was reading at the second or third grade level, they passed me from eighth grade.

My sixth grade teacher was the only teacher who said I should have my hearing checked. The seventh and eighth grade teachers didn't care, or if they did, they certainly didn't show it. They just let me sit in the classroom and do nothing. I resent that, because in high school I had to start all over to get the basics I had missed. My high school teachers were pretty good.

Tina Priest:

I didn't have any bad elementary teachers. My worst high school teacher was deaf and couldn't communicate with the students. Her sign language was awful and she talked down to us. She was very boring.

Lulu Sinsabaugh:

I had one English teacher I didn't like very much in high school. His attitude was not very good. He thought he knew so much more than anybody else. He was very intelligent, but he couldn't relate very well to the students.

Roxanne Ruiz:

I had a junior high school teacher I didn't like very much. If I made one little mistake, she would go crazy. Sometimes she would yell at me. I think she wanted to strangle me sometimes!

Shannon Kidder:

In elementary school, I remember one teacher would scare us because she would get really mad. For example, if a student wasn't paying attention she would go over and grab the student, and then drag him over to a corner of the room.

In high school, I had a math teacher that would not talk about math and rarely wrote on the board. He seemed to expect the students to understand about math by themselves. When you asked him to explain something, he wouldn't explain it very well. He wasted the students' time.

Debbie Pruett:

My elementary school teachers were pretty good.

I had a deaf high school teacher who liked to tell jokes. He wasted too much time. I learned very little from him.

Lori Little:

My elementary school teachers were pretty good, but a couple in high school were not too good. I had a deaf science teacher who was super boring. She killed all enthusiasm for learning about science. She talked baby talk to the students.

Another deaf high school teacher would frequently insult the students. He would hurt their feelings. He always seemed to be talking in negatives.

Jenny Simpson:

I remember one teacher I had when I was seven years old. She would really yell at the students when they didn't pay attention. If one student was caught talking to another student, she would slap the student's hand with a ruler. She was a mean teacher.

The high school teachers I didn't like were those who would bring their own problems into the classroom. Sometimes they would yell at the students for no apparent reason. They should have left their personal problems at home.

Some of the other high school teachers would bother me when they showed no patience. Sometimes I just didn't understand.

What is the best way to communicate with a deaf child?

Tami Saddler:
Total Communication.

John Saddler:
And make sure you include the oral as well as the manual parts of that program!

Tina Priest:
If the child has enough hearing to develop speech and will be able to successfully communicate orally, then by all means emphasize speech development. On the other hand, if there is any chance where this will not be the case, I would use sign language. Using sign language along with speech is fine so long as the speech is there, too. Signs are not going to hurt the development of speech.

I am severely hard of hearing and my son has normal hearing. I talk and sign with him. I sign with him so he can understand what I want, and he signs with me so I can understand what he wants. He is developing speech and learning sign language at the same time - no problem.

Paula Schurz:
Use a lot of speech and a lot of signs. I would want my child to be able to communicate in both worlds. I would want him to be able to sign with my family and the deaf world, and also be able to talk with his hearing relatives and friends.

How would you discipline a deaf child?

Tami Saddler:
I would be more strict with my children than my parents were with me.

John Saddler:
I would try to be more understanding with my child. I would try to talk things over first and only as a last resort would I spank a child. I am not completely convinced that spanking works.

Tami Saddler:
Oh, I think spanking works - you always remember a spanking! After that, all you need is a good stern facial expression. The child will know if he keeps acting up he will get another spanking. For most children the memory and expression are quite sufficient.

Tina Priest:
I would discipline a child the same way as I was disciplined. I would make very sure he knows why he is being disciplined.

Lulu Sinsabaugh:
When he is young, I would spank him when necessary. Later, I would remove his privileges, like the use of the TV for a few days. When the child is older, I would ground him for one or two days. Maybe, for something very bad, I would

ground him for a full week -but I think this type of punishment for a month is too long.

Debbie Pruett:

First, I would explain to him why his behavior is not
acceptable. Second, I would always give him a fair warning,
so that he would have an opportunity to change his behavior. If the message did not get through then I would punish
him. Yelling at a child is enough. I would never hit a child.

Lori Little:

Explain, explain, explain! I would make sure my child
understood clearly why he was being disciplined. Only after
you have taken the time to explain does the punishment
have meaning. I would also explain to him the exact consequences of bad behavior.

If he were a little stubborn, I would ground him until he
accepted the rules and/or until he apologized for his behavior. That would apply even if he got involved in drugs and
ended up in jail. Assuming I had told him to stay clear of
drugs and he got himself into jail, he would have to rely on
his own resources to get out. I would not come down and
post his bail. It sounds tough, but the consequences had
been explained to him beforehand.

Do you prefer to date hearing people or deaf people?

John Saddler:

The personality is all that matters to me.

Tami Saddler:

I would not date a hearing person. He would not understand my world. I dated a hearing person for four years. He did not accept me for what I was.

Any meaningful relationship involves communication. That was our biggest problem. He would criticize me for not learning how to read lips. I would complain that he would not make the effort to learn sign language.

He wanted me to go to his parties. I didn't want to go because I couldn't be a part of them. I couldn't hear. He thought I was boring because I didn't want to party.

I also would have reservations about dating a deaf person who communicated only through sign language. I would be afraid that he would be too dependent on me. I don't want the burden of someone relying on me for communication with the hearing world. I don't think he would understand my world either. I am hard of hearing, not deaf.

John Saddler:

I would prefer dating a hearing person rather than a deaf person. I am afraid I would be bored with the typical language level of many deaf individuals. Intellectual companionship is very important to me in any relationship I have.

I am not saying a typical deaf person is slow. I am saying a person's language level has to be quite high for me to be content. I think a relatively small percentage of the deaf population has attained that level.

Tina Priest:

It depends upon the individual. He has to be willing to talk slowly and have patience when I don't understand what he is saying.

He would have to realize that I have a hard time going to parties where there is a lot of noise. At those functions it is hard for me to understand individual conversations. I am lost in groups of more than four or five people.

Dating deaf men is a little easier because of the communication factor. We can use sign language and that helps a lot.

Lulu Sinsabaugh:

(Laughter.) You mean if I was not married? I really don't think I would enjoy dating a man with normal hearing. I would not feel totally comfortable. The same would be true for a hard of hearing man. There would always be doubts about what he was saying or if he was cheating on me. When he would reverse-interpret for me, would the message be the exact truth?

I only dated one hearing boy, and that turned out to be a bad experience. He cheated on me a lot. One experience like that was enough! I would prefer to date deaf men. I feel I could trust them more.

Roxanne Ruiz:

I would not be comfortable dating a hearing boy. I don't think I would be a good date for him. I think there would be too many problems when we would try to communicate with each other. Maybe for a short while it would be fun, but because of the communication barriers, I don't think it would be a lasting relationship.

Even though I understand a lot of verbal communication, I would want the support of sign language. For that reason, I think I would be more comfortable dating deaf boys who used sign language. My first choice would be a person who uses both speech and signs.

Paula Schurz:

I would be uncomfortable dating a hearing man who did not know signs. The communication problems would be just too difficult. I don't really feel I would be able to trust him.

I would date deaf men because I would assume the communication problem would be minimal. A deaf man would already know sign language. Actually, I think I would prefer to date a hearing impaired man that was skilled in both signs and speech. I feel I could trust him more.

Shannon Kidder:

It depends upon the personality of the hearing person. If he is sweet, helpful and really cares, then I would be happy to date him. The same is true for the deaf person. The personality of the person is what is most important to me.

I must admit, when I date deaf boys I enjoy it because I can understand all the jokes. I miss that when I date a hearing boy.

Debbie Pruett:

It depends whether I can trust the person. It doesn't make any difference to me if the person is deaf or hearing.

Recently I became a Christian. For a lasting relationship, it would be important to me for the person to feel the same as I do about religion. Then the relationship could be built upon mutual trust and understanding, under God.

Kathy Ferguson:

Though I would date hearing and deaf men, I would prefer to date a hard of hearing man. I think a hard of hearing person would understand my world best. I feel I could trust such a person more. Regardless, I would want a man I was dating either to know sign language or be very willing to learn it.

Lori Little:

I would prefer to date deaf men. I suppose if a hearing man was from a deaf family then I might date him. He would have to know sign language.

Jenny Simpson:

It doesn't make any difference to me if the person is hearing or deaf, but I would want that person to use sign language so he could communicate with me. I would not want to write everything we wanted to say to each other on a piece of paper!

Would you marry a person who had normal hearing?

Tami Saddler:
No, because of the communication problems.

John Saddler:
Yes, I would. It all depends upon the individual.

Tina Priest:
I don't think so. Communication would be too hard. Would my partner be willing to learn sign language and stick to it? Could I really trust him? It would be tough. I think I would be more comfortable with a deaf person.

Roxanne Ruiz:
No way. Too many communication problems. A deaf person who relied totally on signs might be a problem, too. I might get tired of signing all the time!

I would prefer a hard of hearing person. I think that would be the best. He would understand me.

Paula Schurz:
No, there would be too many communication problems. I would marry a deaf person, but I would want him to be able to talk to some extent. Then he would be able to communicate with my family. I guess my first choice would be to marry a hard of hearing person.

Shannon Kidder:

I am not sure I would marry a hearing person. At the very least he would have to know sign language. But if I married someone who had only recently learned sign language, would he still be signing to me three years later? I wonder.

I think I would prefer to marry a hard of hearing person. A hard of hearing person can talk on the telephone, he can interpret, and he also understands deafness.

Debbie Pruett:

Yes, I would marry a hearing person.

Kathy Ferguson:

If the boy could hear, I would want to live with him first to see if we would get along. He would have to use sign language.

I don't think I would be completely comfortable with a deaf man who relied exclusively on signs for communication. Would that be too much for me?

I would prefer to marry a person who was hard of hearing. I think that would be the best.

Lori Little:

If he came from a deaf family and used sign language, I would consider it. If he did not use sign language then I would not marry him. How could we really communicate?

Jenny Simpson:

If the person knew and used sign language, I might marry him. If he did not know it and did not want to learn it, I would not marry him.

The same would be true for a deaf person. He would have to know and use sign language. I do not want to write all my life!

Would it make any difference to you if your children were hearing or deaf?

John Saddler:

It would make no difference to me.

Tami Saddler:

I feel the same.

Tina Priest:

I have a young son who has normal hearing. He is a big help. For instance, he lets me know when someone is at the door or when the telephone is ringing. He is also learning sign language so we will be able to communicate even better as he gets older.

You can get a hearing child's attention by just calling his name. Obviously, that is not the case with a deaf child. You have to go over to a deaf child, take the time to sign, and then make sure he really understands what you are saying. You frequently have a vocabulary as well as a communication barrier to overcome. On the other hand, a deaf child would share my world... I guess it would not make much difference to me whether my child was hearing or deaf.

Lulu Sinsabaugh:

It would not make any difference to me at all. Whether the baby was hearing or deaf, we would teach him sign language because both my husband and I are deaf and that is how we communicate. I don't see any problems either way.

Paula Schurz:

Whether he was deaf or hearing wouldn't matter, because it would be my child.

Shannon Kidder:

It doesn't make any difference to me. I would teach my child sign language so he could communicate with me whether he was hearing or deaf.

If he were hearing he could also interpret for me, though I understand you have to be careful not to give too much interpreting responsibility to a child, especially when he is young.

If he were deaf he would be share my world. In that sense, I would almost prefer deaf children. There might be a closer bond to them.

Kathy Ferguson:

Good question. In a way it would be nice to have deaf children. I think our communication would be quite good because we would rely heavily on sign language. If I were married to a hearing husband and we had hearing children, would they be more likely to talk with him than me?

What would you like to tell teachers of deaf children?

John Saddler:

Treat your deaf students as though they were hearing students. Set high standards. Sure there will be some deaf students who will have more problems than others, but amazing things can happen with proper instruction.

Suppose you have a foreigner who moves to America. Is it right to ask him to come here and get a job without any education or guidance? Teaching him the English language alone will not be sufficient. You also have to teach him American ways in order for him to feel really at home.

The same is true for a deaf person. Having a deaf person find his own way in the hearing world can be very frustrating and confusing. He is like the foreigner. He has to be taught, not only the language, but also the customs in order to really fit in.

The successfulness of a deaf person depends upon each individual. Don't let the lack of motivation of a few reflect upon your feelings toward the rest of the group.

Tami Saddler:

But, John, how can you expect a deaf teacher to teach her students in the same way a hearing teacher teaches her classes? If you are deaf and you have never taught in the hearing schools, how do you know what the instruction standards of the hearing schools are? On top of that, if you as a deaf student attended deaf schools, then when have you ever experienced what hearing schools demand from their students? Think about that.

John Saddler:

Good point. Then to prepare deaf students to compete with their hearing peers, deaf teachers must be made aware of the educational skills their deaf students will be expected to have in the hearing world. If you don't demand as much of deaf students as good schools demand of hearing students, then you have additionally handicapped your deaf students. They will graduate to a very harsh reality.

I feel students have the right to ask for an accounting from their schools and teachers: teachers and school boards set the standards, not the students.

Tami Saddler:

I agree. I have heard rumors that some people are so unhappy with the level of the deaf schools that they advocate closing them down and sending all the students to hearing schools. Some students would be in mainstream situations, and others would be in self-contained classrooms.

I don't think that is the proper solution. A large number of deaf students would not be served appropriately in a mainstream situation. They would miss a lot. They might attend the hearing classes, but they would be lost. Many would actually learn less that way.

Tina Priest:

Use lots of gestures and move. Try to be exciting. Don't have a lot of boring lectures. Involve your students.

Lulu Sinsabaugh:

Explain things in the easiest way possible. Build concepts in all subjects, one step at a time. Make sure a step is mastered before you go on to the next step. In higher math like algebra, do one step at a time for each line.

Paula Schurz:

Use sign language. Speak clearly. Be sensitive to your deaf students' feelings.

Be aware that the deaf world and the hearing world have different cultures, that they are separate and equal. Hearing teachers in particular should try to learn as much about the deaf culture as possible to understand deaf ways. Understanding sign language does not mean you understand deafness!

Shannon Kidder:

Have patience when your students don't understand. If your students can see that you are willing to repeat things for them, they will want to learn from you. If you don't show any patience, then they will feel you don't care about them, and will tune you out.

At the same time, don't repeat things too much. Some teachers say the same thing over and over again. I get so tired of that! Know when to move on.

Debbie Pruett:

Realize that deaf students are individuals. Even within a small group or class the range of abilities can be considerable.

Try to learn about deafness. What are the strengths and weaknesses of this handicap? One of the weaknesses is making many mistakes. Until the concept is completely clear, the individual is going to make a lot of mistakes. Have patience. Work on the weakness until it becomes a strength. Don't give up.

Kathy Ferguson:
Be flexible. You are dealing with individuals.

Lori Little:
Use lots of concrete examples for what you are trying to say. Use lots of encouragement. Ask questions, not only about academics, but what your students think and feel. Make them a part of your class. Talk with the kids, don't just lecture - that will put your students to sleep.

Jenny Simpson:
Don't be afraid to repeat things for those students who aren't getting the message. Keep trying.

Any closing remarks to hearing people?

John Saddler:
Please don't judge a person by the handicap.

Tami Saddler:
Please don't be afraid to teach and communicate with the deaf. They are people with the same wishes, hopes, and fears as you.

Tina Priest:
With my hearing aid, I can hear a lot of what you say. I can fill in a lot by reading your lips. If you show me the courtesy of facing me directly and talking clearly, I can and would like to communicate with you.

Some deaf people do not hear at all and are not skilled in reading lips. Please have patience with them when they ask you to write out your message.

Though some things are different, we are the same in many ways. We have feelings just like you. We have the same frustrations in life that you have. We have our happy times and our sad times.

Shannon Kidder:
Because I am completely deaf, there will be times I will not understand what you are saying to me. When that happens, please do not make a face at me. Have the patience to simply repeat what you said.

Lori Little:

Please don't waste my time with stupid questions. If you are curious about meeting deaf people and want to communicate with us, it would really help to learn sign language.

Jenny Simpson:

Use sign language and have patience when we don't understand. Please realize that deaf people have a wide range of abilities. The language levels of deaf people vary widely. We do not hear the English language, so we miss out on a lot of sentence structure and idioms.

Any closing remarks to parents whose children are deaf?

John Saddler:

Don't treat them any differently than you would hearing children.

Tami Saddler:

Don't limit them. Let them try to do anything they want. If they fail, fine, but at least give them the opportunity to try.

Don't allow your children to use the handicap of not being able to hear as an excuse for not doing things. With some things that may apply, be sensitive to that, but keep the handicap in perspective.

Tina Priest:

Have patience with them. Learn sign language so you can communicate with them. Take the time to involve them in family matters. Take them with you when you go places. Don't leave them out.

Shannon Kidder:

Take the time to explain to them what is happening, particularly those things that involve the family. Do what is necessary to develop your deaf child's pride in himself. Instill a sense of self-worth.

Debbie Pruett:

Learn sign language. Whereas a hearing child absorbs a lot (including language and speech development) by listening to what is going on, a deaf child must be actively taught all of these things.

You can not expect the school to be able to teach your child everything. You will have to become teachers yourselves.

Lori Little:

Treat them the way you would treat hearing children. Encourage them in the same way as you would hearing children. Discipline them in the same way as you would hearing children.

Jenny Simpson:

Don't be afraid to send your child to a deaf school, but closely monitor her progress to see whether she is being challenged. If she is not, then try a hearing school.

Show a lot of patience with your deaf child. Be careful to strike a balance between helping your deaf child and making her too dependent upon you. People with good intentions will often do things for me that I can do for myself. I appreciate their efforts and thoughtfulness, but though I have some limitations, I am not helpless. Like most people, I want to be independent. Are you helping me in the short run but hindering me in the long run?

Encourage your deaf child to grow and have the desire to accomplish things. There is great satisfaction in achieving goals. Allow your deaf child opportunities to reach his goals and foster pride in himself.

Anything else you would like to add?

Paula Schurz:[29]

If parents have deaf children, they (the children) needs a lot of attention from parents to teach or give more love and closer to their family. Not to even to leave them out and not to treat badly if it is innocence.

(Deaf) children needs more love and sharing with their family as playful as they go to Golf'n Stuff or Skateland, etc. So the children would not feel more lonesome or hurt a lot from them. It would raise their (children's) life greatly with the family.

Debbie Pruett:

Deafness is a deeper handicap than most people realize. When many people see deaf people using sign language, they think they see two people who are like them, just that they are communicating with their hands and have a hearing problem.

There is a much greater difference than that between the hearing and deaf worlds. There is not only a language difference, there is also a cultural difference. Perceptions are different.

I think it is wonderful when I see hearing people who are learning sign language. The deaf would love to share their world with you. But please realize that one does not understand deafness just by learning sign language.

Also, please do not be too quick to announce what is best for the deaf if you do not really understand the deaf environ-

---

[29]I have left Paula Schurz's final comment unedited to give the reader its full impact and tenor. The words in parenthesis were added for clarification purposes.

ment. To understand it you have to spend time in our world and learn our culture.

"The deaf" is not one entity: each deaf person has his or her own perspectives, abilities, and skills. Please be cautious in classifying "the deaf."

Do learn sign language, and let us share with each other the insights and perspectives we both have to offer!

IN CLOSING

I hope this book has helped those involved with the hearing impaired. There are many ideas covered here.

A hearing impaired child is first of all a child. Accepting the whole child, hearing loss and all, relieves everybody. Denying the hearing loss and trying to force the child to "become hearing" serves no one. Forget the "Why?" Face the facts, find ways to minimize the loss, and move on.

This is a hearing problem, not a mental problem. Don't be intimidated. Break down the barriers to communication. Auditory stimulation through hearing aids, along with intensive vocabulary and language development is critical. If sign language will help, use it.

Parents are the key. An active ongoing commitment to your child's education will be required if your child is to approach the academic standards of his hearing peers. Become involved. Get with other parents. Share your mutual experiences and concerns with them. Support each other.

If you treat your hearing impaired child in a normal fashion, with the same standards as you would demand from hearing children, then your hearing impaired child will absorb these standards. One handicap is enough. You are not doing your child any favors by lowering standards, whether they are disciplinary or academic.

Be sensitive to your child's frustrations. Hearing aids, while helpful, have many limitations. Especially during the time of adolescence be patient. Over time your child will find a vocation and achievement level that he is most comfortable with. Accept that and everybody will be much happier.

Be prepared for the withdraw symptoms one sometimes sees, not only in adolescence, but also in older people. Be patient. Understand this withdraw is not by choice, but only to shield oneself from embarrassment.

You are not alone. The more you learn about hearing loss, the less of a mystery it is. You will become more confident, and will realize that a hearing impairment can be dealt with successfully.

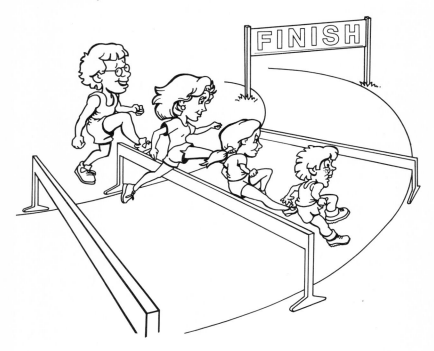

APPENDIX

Organizations that offer services and support:

Self Help for the Hard of Hearing (SHHH)
7800 Wisconsin Avenue
Bethesda, Maryland 20814

Alexander Graham Bell Association for the Deaf
3417 Volta Place, N.W.
Washington, D.C. 20007
Phone: (202) 337-5220

American Association of Late Deafened Adults
1027 Oakton
Evanston, Ill. 60202

John Tracy Clinic
806 West Adams Blvd.
Los Angeles, Ca. 90007
Phone: (213) 748-5481 Voice / (213) 747-2924 TDD

Tripod
2901 N. Keystone Street
Burbank, Ca. 91504

American Society for Deaf Children
814 Thayer Avenue
Silver Spring, Maryland 20910
Phone: (301) 585-5400 Voice or TDD

Convention of the American Instructors for the Deaf
P.O. Box 2025
Austin, Texas 78768
Phone: (512) 441-2225 Voice or TDD

National Association of the Deaf
814 Thayer Avenue
Silver Spring, Maryland 20910
Phone: (301) 587-1733 Voice or TDD

National Information Center on Deafness
800 Florida Avenue, N.E.
Washington, D.C. 20002-3625

Harc Mercantile, Ltd.
P.O. Box 3055
Kalamazoo, Michigan 49003-3055

Sunburst Communications
101 Castleton Street
Pleasantville, N.Y. 10570
Phone: (800) 431-1934